Praise for *Heavy Flow*

Reading *Heavy Flow* is akin to a long chat with a non-judgmental super cool big sister who knows her stuff. Grounded in a fierce feminist commitment to body literacy as an act of resistance, Laird guides the reader toward better health and body positivity without the saccharine. Readable, inclusive, real, and often funny, *Heavy Flow* is a myth-busting manual and menstrual cycle roadmap that insists menstruators be seen and heard.

— Chris Bobel, author of *The Managed Body: Developing Girls and Menstrual Health in the Global South* and *New Blood: Third Wave Feminism and the Politics of Menstruation*

Heavy Flow breaks down absolutely everything you need to know about menstruation. Expertly written and easy to understand, this book takes the shame out of menstruation and empowers women to feel great about their bodies.

— Ariel Ng Bourbonnais, author and co-editor of *Through, Not Around* and co-founder of The 16 Percent

As fierce as it is fascinating, *Heavy Flow* outlines the path of the pro-period movement, bringing that red wave right up to your own front door and the reader's personal period experience. What could this cultural moment mean for you and your reproductive health? Laird answers this question with confidence and compassion, skillfully translating the hashtags into clear, honest, and much needed health information. This is one of those books that's going to be hard to keep to yourself — you'll be loaning it out and losing it to your best friend, your sister, your daughter.

— Holly Grigg-Spall, author of *Sweetening the Pill: Or How We Got Hooked on Hormonal Birth Control*

Heavy Flow is an important addition to the global conversation about periods. Periods are coming out in the open more than ever before, and as more women discover the connection between healthy menstrual cycles and overall health, they need a place to turn for guidance. Amanda has put together an encouraging and easily accessible resource for women as they strive for better periods. Amanda's passion for demystifying the menstrual cycle and eradicating menstrual taboos shines through on every page!

— Lisa Hendrickson-Jack, fertility awareness educator and author of *The Fifth Vital Sign: Master Your Cycles and Optimize Your Fertility*

Amanda demystifies menstruation for us in a way that is eye-opening and fascinating. I felt excited reading her book knowing that many women will have access to this information and will be able to take charge of their own hormonal health and bleed with awareness! I sure wish I had this information when I was popping the birth control pill for over a decade.

— Joy McCarthy, CNP, best-selling author of *Joyous Health and Joyous Detox*

Somehow Amanda Laird makes the "curse" of menstruation almost feel like a blessing. She's written an incredibly thoughtful and informative guide to not only understanding your body better, but also learning how to have deeper compassion for it, too. Required reading for every person that has (or ever will) experience the "flow."

— Jessica Murnane, author of *One Part Plant* and founder of Know Your Endo

Heavy Flow delivers the goods: Amanda Laird gives the menstrual lowdown about why we don't have to keep periods on the downlow. I love how she consistently challenges corporate messages of shame and shares her own personal, professional, and practical ideas while effortlessly introducing stuff from the wider menstrual research community. It's all done with a fun and enthusiastic push toward body literacy and empowerment; readers will feel like they're part of the podcast or hanging out with a friend. It's very period positive and it's a welcome addition to the growing global period library. I'm so glad it's here!

— Chella Quint, comedian, artist, menstruation education researcher, and
#periodpositive founder

Heavy Flow is the book I wish I had when I was a teenager and am glad to have now. Amanda Laird answers questions you didn't even know you had about the menstrual cycle with topics ranging from political relevance, to practical physiology, to nutritional support for people who menstruate.

— Kathleen Shannon, creative entrepreneur, author, and speaker

Heavy Flow is essential reading for all menstruators. Laird challenges readers to think about their period in broader feminist terms, including that women's pain is too often dismissed, and how essential menstrual products are out of reach for many. I look forward to having a copy on the shelf of our wellness centre.

— Caroline Starr, co-director of The Healing Collective, author and co-editor of
Through, Not Around, and co-founder of The 16 Percent

HEAVY FLOW.

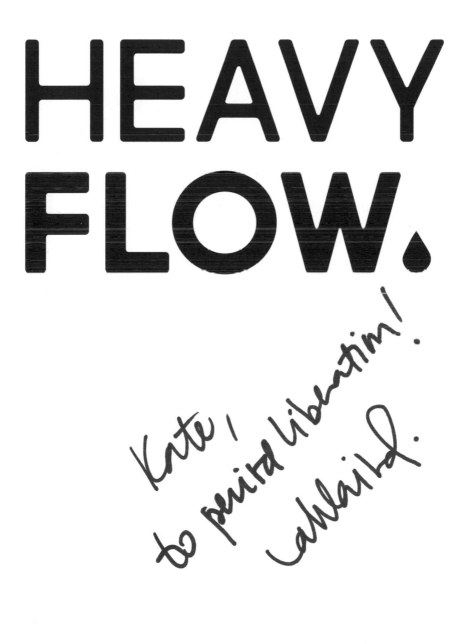

Kate,

to period liberation!

Amanda Laird.

HEAVY FLOW.

BREAKING THE CURSE
OF MENSTRUATION

AMANDA LAIRD

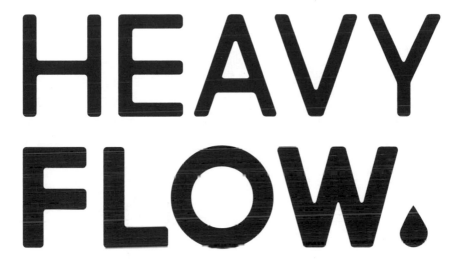

DUNDURN
TORONTO

Cover design: Laura Boyle
Printer: Webcom, a division of Marquis Printing Inc.

Library and Archives Canada Cataloguing in Publication

Laird, Amanda, author
        Heavy flow : breaking the curse of menstruation / Amanda
Laird.

Includes bibliographical references and index.
Issued in print and electronic formats.
ISBN 978-1-4597-4313-7 (softcover).--ISBN 978-1-4597-4314-4
(PDF).--ISBN 978-1-4597-4315-1 (EPUB)

        1. Menstruation--Social aspects. 2. Women--Health and
hygiene--Social aspects. I. Title.

GN484.38.L35 2019   612.6'62   C2018-906290-8
                                            C2018-906291-6

1 2   3   4   5   23 22   21   20   19

 Conseil des Arts   Canada Council
du Canada   for the Arts

We acknowledge the support of the **Canada Council for the Arts**, which last year invested $153 million to bring the arts to Canadians throughout the country, and the **Ontario Arts Council** for our publishing program. We also acknowledge the financial support of the **Government of Ontario**, through the **Ontario Book Publishing Tax Credit** and **Ontario Creates**, and the **Government of Canada**.

Nous remercions le **Conseil des arts du Canada** de son soutien. L'an dernier, le Conseil a investi 153 millions de dollars pour mettre de l'art dans la vie des Canadiennes et des Canadiens de tout le pays.

Care has been taken to trace the ownership of copyright material used in this book. The author and the publisher welcome any information enabling them to rectify any references or credits in subsequent editions.

                                                                — J. Kirk Howard, President

The publisher is not responsible for websites or their content unless they are owned by the publisher.

Printed and bound in Canada.

VISIT US AT

🏛 dundurn.com | 🐦 @dundurnpress | f dundurnpress | 📷 dundurnpress

Dundurn
3 Church Street, Suite 500
Toronto, Ontario, Canada
M5E 1M2

Dedicated to everyone on their period
— yesterday, today, and tomorrow —
especially Maisie Clementine.

Only once we are educated about our cycles and the cultural associations can we recognize it for what it really is: not a shameful secret but a fact of life that need not be concealed.

— Elizabeth Kissling, *Capitalizing on the Curse:*
The Business of Menstruation

CONTENTS

PART 3: EMBRACING YOUR CYCLE

INTRODUCTION

I was, somewhat ironically, in health class when it happened. I didn't even have to look to know what was happening — the telltale warmth spreading from between my legs told me exactly what I needed to know.

My pad was leaking.

I excused myself from the classroom, tucked a fresh pad into the sleeve of my sweater and stealthily inspected the chair I had been sitting on to make sure there was no blood on it. Thankfully, there was not — my classmates were *still* talking about the girl who stained a chair the term before. I shuffled my way to the washroom, keeping my legs tightly crossed to avoid another gush of blood and any further leakage.

Sure enough, I had soaked through my pad and stained both my underwear and my jeans. I changed into a fresh pad, but the damage was done — the blood was visible on the outside. Mortified, I spent the rest of the day with my winter jacket tied around my waist. While the bloodstain had been concealed, the jacket-around-the-waist trick was pretty much like sending out a bat signal to every other student in my school that my pad had leaked.

Does this sound like a familiar story? I'm sure anyone reading this book has a period horror story of their own; whether it's the classic leaky pad in middle school, a bloodstain on the sheets of a new lover's bed, or a tampon rolling out of your bag at the most inopportune time. Having someone know you're on your period — or worse, actually seeing the blood evidence — is embarrassing.

Or maybe your period horror story doesn't have to do with a bloodstain, but the pain that is often experienced with menstruation. Period pain is real pain, and it's estimated that it affects anywhere from 70 percent to 90 percent of people who menstruate.

That's a hell of a lot of "bad periods," a term that Meghan Cleary, founder of the aptly named resource website Bad-Periods.com, defines as "a condition enshrined in mystery, myth, cultural shame, taboo and clinical gender bias."

Never mind *bad* periods: all periods are enmeshed in the same issues. Full stop.

Despite all our advances as a species, menstruation is something that remains a relative mystery for many humans. We can put a man on the moon, yet almost half of the world's population is suffering on a monthly basis, often in silence, because of a perfectly natural bodily function. Menstrual cramps are the most common gynecological problem in adolescent girls[1] and are the leading cause of short-term absences from school and work.

In a 1978 essay for *Ms.* magazine, Gloria Steinem mused that if men could menstruate, "Congress would fund a National Institute of Dysmenorrhea to help stamp out monthly discomforts." Steinem adds that if men could menstruate they would brag about how long and how much, and menstrual products would be free. For anyone who has ever had a period, the essay is hilarious, but it's also a bleak commentary on the ways in which menstruation is used as a tool of the patriarchy.

More than forty years later, Steinem's missive is still relevant.

No such pain institute has been founded, and the options for managing period pain and other related symptoms are still limited — and many have to spend years convincing doctors to take that pain seriously.

We live in a culture that seems to have no taboos left, yet period shame still persists. In a world where the minutiae of our lives are live-tweeted, posted to Instagram, and enshrined online, we wouldn't dare update our status to "menstruating."

And menstrual products certainly aren't free. In fact, quite the opposite — for some they can be downright expensive. The "feminine hygiene" industry brings in about $15 billion in sales worldwide; that figure doesn't include pain medication and other sundries related to menstruation. There are many people around the world who simply cannot afford to purchase pads or tampons, or don't have access to them in remote areas, relying instead on rags, grass, newspaper, scraps of fabric, or even cow dung to manage their flow. These found materials are itchy, unhygienic, and unreliable. Rather than risk the shame of having their menstruation exposed, many girls and women simply stay home from school and work.

It's nothing short of a human rights violation. If that sounds extreme, the United Nations Human Rights Council says the same thing in no uncertain terms: "The lack of access to adequate water and sanitation services, including menstrual hygiene management, and *the widespread stigma associated with menstruation, have a negative impact on gender equality and the human rights of women and girls.*"[2] (emphasis mine)

During my career as a nutritionist, I've developed an interest in menstrual cycles from a health perspective. Although I had a lifelong interest in reproductive health, even sewing my own pads and making zines about toxic ingredients in tampons while I was in high school, I was almost thirty before I learned about how my menstrual cycle really worked and that it was a vital sign, both a promoter and indicator of good health. It wasn't until I was in nutrition school that I was presented with the idea that period pain wasn't "normal."

As a feminist, I see that menstruation is a complex issue that transcends physiology. The more time I spend writing, reading, and researching menstruation, the more I recognize just how far the influence of the menstrual taboo reaches. It's entwined with feminism and patriarchy, gender and the rights of trans people.

Follow the red thread and you will uncover how the medical system's paternalistic, "doctor knows best" approach has not just ignored, but denied the pain of so many for centuries and has literally failed women by leaving them out of medical and drug trials because controlling the menstrual cycle is, well, hard — 80 percent of the prescription drugs pulled from the U.S. market between 1997 and 2001 caused more side effects in women than in men.[3]

Go a little farther and you'll see how menstruation is a sister to the conversation around hormonal birth control; cousin to female sexuality, fertility, pregnancy, and abortion. It's about what we as a society think is okay to do to female bodies.

Menstruation intersects with capitalism, the illusion of consumer choice, and the role that product manufacturers have played in shaping the mainstream conversation around menstruation, for worse *and* for better.

It is at once a political issue, a cultural issue, a class issue, and a public health issue. Our attitudes toward menstruation mirror our discomfort with seasonality and change, death and renewal. It's underpinned by centuries of shame and taboo, fear and reverence, misunderstanding and symbolism.

No wonder they call it "The Curse."

Yet, I believe the curse can be broken.

Elizabeth Kissling, author of *Capitalizing on the Curse: The Business of Menstruation*, wrote that menstruation will no longer be a curse only when women determine how they relate to their menstrual cycles on their own terms. This book is a guide to understanding your menstrual cycle and claiming this vital sign — on your own terms.

The first step in breaking the curse is unpacking the centuries of shame and taboo that have kept menstruation a mystery to both menstruators and medical professionals, which we will do in the following pages, before we get to the meat of it. In part one, you'll find a back-to-basics, 101-style guide to understanding your menstrual cycle and moving toward body literacy. Then, in part two, I will present the practical applications for improving your menstrual experience, including how to practise self-advocacy within the conventional medical system; the benefits of working with paramedical and alternative health practitioners; and how to use food to have a better period. The final section of this book is dedicated to the different ways that you can explore embracing your period in a way that feels meaningful to you, and how to talk to the next generation to make sure that the shame stops here.

A note about language. At times this book uses binary terms such as women and men, if only to highlight how the experiences and representations of women specifically differ, particularly within medicine, from that of men. I recognize that not everyone who identifies as a woman menstruates, and that not everyone who menstruates identifies as a woman, and as such, I use inclusive language when discussing the physical process of menstruation.

A SHORT HISTORY OF THE CURSE

That time when my pad leaked in health class, I hadn't even had my period for a full year. And yet, I knew intrinsically that it was something that I needed to hide; that if anyone saw the blood that had soaked through and stained my jeans, it would have been the ultimate embarrassing moment. Social suicide. Death by period stain.

"Even if it was your worst enemy in high school, even if it was that popular girl that was always mean to you, if she bled through her jeans you would tell her," said Abby Norman, author of *Ask Me About My Uterus*. "That is ultimate girl code; that is the worst thing that could ever happen to somebody."[1]

It's that embarrassment that makes you tuck a tampon up your sleeves on the way to the bathroom or to buy the crinkle-free pads that are designed for utter discretion in public restrooms. One company even designed a new tampon that would fit in the palm of your hand to ensure that it wouldn't be seen on your way to the bathroom. It's what makes us opt for odour-free protection and talk in euphemisms like "It's that time of the month" or "Aunt Flow is on her way," instead of just saying "I'm menstruating."

By another name, it's shame.

Brené Brown, a renowned shame researcher and author of several books on the subject, defines shame as the intensely painful feeling or experience of believing that we are flawed and therefore unworthy of love and belonging — something we've experienced, done, or failed to do makes us unworthy of connection.[2]

When it comes to menstrual shame, the thing that you've "done" to make you unworthy is a perfectly natural bodily process. Shame is born from the idea that menstrual blood, and in turn menstruating bodies, is gross, dirty, and disgusting.

If you've ever spent time with a young child, you know that shame isn't something we're born with; it's impressed upon us by external influences such as social norms and structures. We are taught to be ashamed. I look at my daughter, who's just three years old, how she moves about the world as if it truly is her oyster — particularly when she's naked, especially when she's naked and wearing her Elsa cape. She is beautifully, wonderfully free of any shame about her body or its functions — because she hasn't yet learned to feel shame about them.

There's nothing inherently shameful about menstruation. It's a perfectly normal, healthy function of a body — tissue mixed with blood and mucus, exiting the body. The shame, along with the stigma and taboos of menstruation, is something we learn along the way, often before we've even reached menarche, the first menstruation. We might first hear about "the curse" from our mothers or sisters, or from older girls in higher grades, whispering on the school playground. We learn about menstruation through the lens of advertising on TV, in magazines, product placement, and online, where it is rarely, if ever, mentioned in a positive light. The rare reference to menstruation in pop culture is usually a punchline, an excuse for a female character's bitchy behaviour or the reason why she turned down sex.

Billion-dollar companies that profit from the shame and disgust that we associate with periods, vaginas, and female sexuality reinforce many of today's menstrual myths. In fact, much of the mainstream narrative about menstruation is funded by corporations. How many of us learned about menstruation from product marketing? Both online and in the classroom, these same companies fund puberty education programs, shaping attitudes — and ensuring brand loyalty — from our very first interactions with menstruation, often before our bodies have matured. It's likely that you didn't even realize that your sex education class was sponsored content.

Menstruation is such a taboo topic that the only acceptable time to discuss it is within the context of products and how to manage it. From the companies that manufacture conventional pads and tampons made with harmful ingredients, to pharmaceutical companies peddling hormonal contraception, people are getting rich off the shame, taboo, and misinformation associated with menstruation.

Manufacturers of menstrual products drive much of the mainstream narrative around menstruation through advertising and marketing, often cleverly discussed as "education." Disposable pads were introduced to the mass market in the 1920s. By the 1930s, product manufacturers began publishing educational leaflets to teach girls about the menstrual cycle. In the absence of widespread reproductive health education, these pamphlets were important. They were also a convenient way to reinforce product marketing messages.

As communications channels moved online in the nineties, companies established educational websites to provide adolescents with information about their changing bodies, and, conveniently, the products available for purchase to manage them.

Procter & Gamble, the makers of Always and Tampax, provide North American schools with free puberty education toolkits. The cleverly on-brand Always Changing® program includes toolkits for teachers, printed materials, and a demonstration kit that includes samples of deodorant and "feminine products," to help teachers "effectively teach in the classroom." In the booklets, which are gender-specific and make no mention of what puberty means for the other sex, kids are taught the basic facts about the changes happening in their body and are also given tips for general good hygiene, managing new body odours, dealing with acne, shaving, "vaginal discharge," and how to choose menstrual products.[3]

Among the products sold in the P&G family of companies are deodorant, disposable razors, tampons, pads, panty liners, toothpaste, face wash, soap, and shampoo.

There's no argument that adolescents need to be educated about menstruation, puberty, and the changes happening in their bodies. And certainly, there are good health reasons for bathing regularly and managing period blood. However, the waters are muddied when education mixes with commerce. Make no mistake: companies that are printing free literature, building websites, and providing educational materials and samples in schools aren't doing it out of the goodness of their hearts. They are building life long brand loyalty.

Beyond education tools, menstrual product advertisements rarely, if ever, paint menstruation in a positive light. Instead, ads focus on concealment, stressing that leak-free, odour-free *protection* is of utmost importance.

Protection from what? The shame of someone finding out you're on your period?

The "menstrual hygiene" industry has a vested interest in your period shame. They're the ones reinforcing taboos by telling you that you need to hide your yucky period — which, by the way, is so offensive it can't even be shown on TV or in print advertising and is instead depicted with a mysterious blue liquid (if your period is blue, skip right ahead to the "what does a normal period look like" section of this book). These same companies are the ones conveniently also selling the products you need to keep your period out of sight and out of mind.

But the makers of Tampax or Always didn't invent period shame as a way to sell their products; they've simply built the growing worldwide "femmecare" industry by capitalizing on centuries of taboo.

EARLY MENSTRUAL MYTHS

From the earliest writings about medicine and physiology, menstruation has been viewed as a mysterious, at times magical, bodily function: something that clearly differentiates female bodies from male. Not only did women bleed and not die from menstrual blood, they did it again about a moon's cycle later. Early people probably noticed that the bleeding stopped with pregnancy. Menstruation's association with creation meant that it was powerful, perhaps even divine, ensuring that it was met with both fear and reverence.

By 77 AD, Pliny the Elder, a Roman author and naval commander, had this to say about menstruation in his thirty-seven-volume tome *Natural History* — the book about practically anything and everything: "Contact with the monthly flux of women turns new wine sour, crops touched by it become barren, rats die, seeds in gardens are dried up, the fruit of trees fall off, the edge of steel and the gleam of ivory are dulled, hives of bees die, even bronze and iron are at once seized by rust, and a horrible smell fills the air; to taste it drives dogs mad and infects their bites with an incurable poison."[4]

At the same time, Pliny also wrote that the antidote to crop failure was to have a menstruating woman walk naked through the field, given that menstrual blood had fertilizing properties. In many societies menstrual blood emits a mana, a supernatural or magical power, and is often associated with fertility.

These opposing views highlight the paradox of menstrual blood. Is menstrual blood dangerous or sacred? Does it create or destroy? Either way, it was clearly regarded as pretty powerful stuff.

Early menstrual taboos affected mealtimes, bedtimes, hunting season ... you know, the times and places where women mingled with men. Menstruating women were not allowed to use the same utensils or share mealtimes with their families; they were not allowed to enter places of worship and were relegated to sleeping in menstrual huts. Intercourse while menstruating was strictly forbidden as it was believed this would have an effect on the hunt.

Taboos exist to protect human beings from danger. Menstrual taboos are practices that help others to avoid a menstruating woman and her dangerous influence, perhaps enabling her to get through her period without succumbing to her own deadly power. One thing is clear: these taboos seem to protect *men* from the mysterious substance of menstruation more than the menstruating woman herself.

Much of the fear and mysticism that has surrounded menstruation for centuries is the result of our limited understanding of how the body works. In Pliny's era, we didn't know much about any bodies, not just female bodies and menstruation.

But even as medical science advanced, female bodies were seen as a deformity of the male body or flat-out ignored — right up until the early 1990s, when, at last, it was mandated that women had to be included in research studies and clinical drug trials.

The ancient Greek philosopher Aristotle believed that menstruation was a sign of a women's inferiority and looked at the female state as a deformity of the male body, which was believed to be the "correct" form for the human body. He believed that menstrual blood was the matter of creation, and that it needed to mix with sperm in order to form a baby. Not a bad guess, really. However, Aristotle saw the female role in reproduction as passive, bringing the physical matter needed to form a human to the party. Males contributed the soul, the more important part of the human body, through their sperm.

Later doctors and philosophers believed that women simply had too much blood and their poorly constructed, inferior female bodies weren't able to keep it all in.

Regnier de Graaf, a seventeenth-century physician, wrote that menstrual blood "escapes by the feeblest parts of the body, in the same way that wine or beer undergoing fermentation escapes by defective parts of the barrel."[5]

The "plethora theory" that women simply had too much blood held up for centuries. It paired well with humorism, an early system of medicine adopted by Ancient Greek and Roman philosophers that detailed the makeup and workings of the human body through four distinct bodily fluids, known as humours. These humours — blood, phlegm, yellow bile, and black bile — and an excess or deficiency of any of these influenced a person's temperament and health.

By the nineteenth century, doctors had begun to question various aspects of the plethora theory as medicine moved away from the humours model of bodily regulation and began to connect menstruation more closely with ovulation, theorizing that menstrual bleeding was similar to the estrus bleeding dogs experience when in heat. Women bled because they were fertile, and therefore were at their sexual peak during that time. While the period-sex taboo has complex origins — we'll come back to that one later — it seems rather convenient that sex would be considered most taboo at the exact time a woman's sexual interest was believed to be highest.

Menstrual blood was often believed to be noxious right up to the twentieth century. In 1920, a Viennese researcher published a paper titled "The Menstrual Poison," which detailed several experiments that "proved" that menotoxins in menstrual blood killed flowers and would inhibit the rising of bread dough. An experiment at Harvard University in 1952 concluded that menstrual blood contained harmful bacteria when mice injected with menstrual blood died, while those injected with a mix of menstrual blood and antibiotics did not. Further studies were unable to replicate these findings.

Another recent misunderstanding of the purpose of menstruation was put forth by Margie Profet, a controversial evolutionary biologist, who published an article in the *Quarterly Review of Biology* in 1993 that theorized that menstruation existed as a way to rid the female body of disease brought in by men's sperm. This theory found little support in experiments or among the scientific community.[6]

Even today, why we menstruate when other large mammals reabsorb the lining of the uterus remains a relative mystery.

THE MODERN MENSTRUAL TABOO

Although these theories have all been disproved or debunked, the idea that menstrual blood is dirty, poisonous, or toxic is still pervasive. I'm often asked when teaching workshops if menstrual blood is the "same" as the blood in the rest of our bodies. Many participants are surprised to learn that it is not, in fact, a toxic substance.

While menstrual theories evolved throughout history as medicine advanced, they all had a common theme: menstruation is a sign of a woman's otherness and her inferiority. Science was used to rationalize her oppression. Menstruation remained a mystery for so long because men didn't menstruate. And perhaps this comes as no surprise: they didn't consider asking women for their perspective on the matter.

Thanks to modern medicine, we now know that menstruation is a part of the menstrual cycle and reproductive system. We know that the uterine lining thickens to prepare for the implantation of a fertilized egg. If no such egg arrives, hormones trigger menstruation — shedding the uterine lining, made up of mucus, blood, and tissue and starting the whole cycle over again. It's clear that menstrual blood is not poison.

However, while we might now have a deeper understanding of reproductive health, this knowledge has not freed us of shame and taboo; menstrual myths are still common today.

Perhaps when you hear "menstrual myth" you think about the various ways that the menstrual taboo has been interpreted in other cultures around the world. For example, in parts of India, women are still barred from entering temples while on their periods, or from touching certain foods. In parts of Africa many believe that it's dangerous for others to see your menstrual blood. And in rural Nepal, many girls and women are still sleeping in menstrual huts — and dying there.[7]

Here in the West, we might be able to move about as we please while menstruating and we're no longer handing over discreet coupons in exchange for menstrual pads to avoid having to ask for them in a drugstore, but we've hardly been liberated from period shame.

In their 1988 book *The Curse: A Cultural History of Menstruation*, co-authors Janice Delaney, Mary Jane Lupton, and Emily Toth write, "Women continue to suffer the taboos of centuries. Law, medicine, religion and psychology have isolated and devalued the menstruating women…. Menstruation is a factor in the control of women by men not only in ancient and primitive societies, where knowledge of physiology is rudimentary at best, but also in our post-industrial world."

It's been thirty years since *The Curse* was published, and like Gloria Steinem's famous essay *If Men Could Menstruate*, it could easily have been written today.

As long as we're still concerning ourselves with concealing menstruation, keeping it a secret, ignoring period pains, having our period pains ignored by doctors, and underestimating the role the menstrual cycle plays in our overall health, we're still in the shackles of the myth.

THE YEAR OF THE PERIOD

In 2015, a number of high-profile, Instagram-worthy events propelled periods out of the stalls of the women's restroom and above the fold in mainstream news outlets and online. NPR dubbed 2015 "The Year of the Period,"[8] while *Cosmopolitan* said it was the year "periods went public."[9]

It all started with an Instagram post.

Early in 2015, artist and poet Rupi Kaur posted a self-portrait on her Instagram account, a not-unusual activity for a young person of the times. In the photo, Kaur is lying on her bed, her back to the camera, which reveals a telltale bloodstain on her grey sweatpants and the sheets. You don't have to think too hard to know what's happening in the scene. The photo was part of a larger series titled "period." What's striking about the images is not that they are remarkable, but quite the opposite — they are intimate and familiar to anyone who has ever had a period. A hot water bottle clutched to an abdomen, a used pad dropped into a wastebasket, a stubborn streak of blood leftover in a toilet bowl.

Instagram not once, but twice removed the photo of Kaur and the bloodstain for violating the social media photo sharing platform's community guidelines — a policy that prohibits photos depicting sex, violence, or nudity. There is nothing explicit in the guidelines about menstrual blood.

In response, Kaur wrote on Facebook, "Thank you Instagram for providing me with the exact response my work was created to critique."[10] The artist statement posted to the website showcasing the "period" photos states that the series was designed to challenge a taboo.[11] The fact that Instagram removed the post proved that it was successful.

What was so offensive about the image of a woman curled up in bed with a period stain on her pants and sheets? At this very moment, about 800 million people on the planet are currently on their periods, making it likely that scenes just like this are playing out in bedrooms all over the world. As anyone who has ever had a period will tell you, blood leaks. Given the innocuous nature of the photo, perhaps it's not the image that was offensive, but simply Kaur's gall to show it in public.

On Instagram, my search for #blood yields 8.4 million results. I find a gallery of images that run the gamut from surgeries to the bloodied faces of UFC fighters, gory special effects makeup, vampires, selfies snapped while giving blood, and a handful of disturbing self-harm images that *do* clearly violate Instagram's community guidelines. In the first couple hundred images that I scroll through, menstruation is noticeably absent, save for a smiling woman holding up a reusable cloth pad. Despite being tagged with #blood, the pad is unused and there is no blood in the picture.

Images of blood dominate mainstream media — in the news, movies, and on television. A massacre at the infamous *Game of Thrones* Red Wedding depicts the brutal murders of several characters, blood spurting, gushing, and leaking all over the screen. By the time it's over, the wedding feast is literally swimming in blood. More than 6.3 million viewers tuned in to watch the episode.[12]

This difference in the way we establish different *kinds* of blood is significant. Breanne Fahs, a professor of Women and Gender Studies at Arizona State University, highlights how blood is gendered in her book *Out for Blood: Essays on Menstruation and Resistance.* Men pass down bloodlines, sacrifice their blood, loose blood in battle and during wars. So, it's not blood that we find offensive, but women's blood and menstrual blood, with its paradoxical association between life and death.

Not long after Kaur's "period" piece made headlines, it was again an image of menstrual blood that propelled Kiran Gandhi, an artist and musician who performs under the moniker Madame Gandhi, onto front pages around the world when she ran the 2015 London Marathon on her period without any menstrual products, opting instead to prioritize her own comfort to "free-bleed," a term coined to describe the act of menstruating right into your clothes instead of using a product to soak it up.

Following the race, Gandhi wrote about the experience on her blog: how it left her feeling empowered and also connected to those women around the world who don't have access to products to manage their flow.

The article, along with the striking photos of Gandhi's bloodstained tights, went viral.

The fact that so much of this conversation centred around the image of a bloodstain and not on the fact that this young woman had just, you know, *run a marathon*, an incredible feat of physical strength, is a perfect example of the period paradox, a term coined by Elizabeth Yuko, bioethicist and writer, in her 2016 essay for *The Establishment* "Period Pain Must Be Taken Seriously — But It Also Shouldn't Define Us."[13] The period paradox ensures that there's no chance of your period holding you back from accomplishing amazing things in your life — just as long as no one has to see it or hear about it.

Menstruation even entered into the U.S. presidential campaign race in 2015 when Donald Trump accused Fox News host Megyn Kelly of having "blood coming out of her wherever."

The events of 2015 launched the term "menstrual equity" into the vernacular, thanks to Jennifer Weiss-Wolf, a lawyer, activist, and author of *Periods Gone Public*. While some North Americans may have been aware of the issue of girls in Africa and Asia missing school because of a lack of access to menstrual products, clean water, and privacy, many of us failed to realize that this was also a domestic issue affecting low-income and homeless people who menstruate in our very own towns and cities. A box of pads or tampons can run anywhere between $5 and $10 — and the heavier your flow or the longer your period is, the more products you need each cycle. When you're on a strict budget, that could mean a choice between food or menstrual products. Faced with that decision, one certainly feels optional compared to the other.

That same year, Canada abolished all taxes on menstrual products in response to the #NoTaxOnTampons campaign created by a group calling themselves The Canadian Menstruators. Even without the tax, however, menstrual products still remain inaccessible to many.

In the U.S., activists began the work to repeal taxes on menstrual products, state by state, and also pushed to increase access to products for those who need them in public spaces such as schools, shelters, and prisons. At the time of writing, just nine states in the U.S. specifically exempt menstrual products from sales tax and another five have legislation pending.[14] In the remaining states, menstrual management products like pads and tampons are often classified as a luxury or non-necessity item. While it varies from state-to-state, a few examples of tax-free necessities include BBQ sunflower seeds, Mardi Gras beads, and — wait for it — Viagra.

When you walk into a public washroom you'll find toilet paper and soap there for you to use. Why? Because it was decided that we all have a right to these items when using the washroom. So why not pads or tampons? Like anything else you do in a public washroom, menstruation is a bodily function that you can't help. Half the population can't help menstruating, yet the products that we need to manage them are taxed, often as luxury items, and kept out of reach for many marginalized individuals who need them. Here in Toronto, where I live, menstrual products aren't even a line item on city-funded shelters, drop-ins, or health centres; although in June 2018 a motion was passed by Toronto's City Council to include tampons and pads in the 2019 budget.

As awareness of "period poverty" has grown, countless menstrual product drives have been set up by student organizations, charities, and NGOs across North America to ensure that people who need them have access to products to manage their periods. This helps, but certainly doesn't solve the problem. Safe, dignified periods are still out of reach for many who menstruate in the world's most affluent countries.

MENSTRUAL ACTIVISM AND PERIOD FEMINISM

So, by now you might be asking yourself, "Where are all the feminists?"

When you start to follow the thread of period shame and taboo, it leads you squarely to patriarchy; yet period poverty and dismantling the menstrual taboos that still exist today are noticeably absent from mainstream feminism — although it had existed "on the wings" for many years before the Year of the Period.

I asked Chris Bobel, author of *New Blood: Third-Wave Feminism and the Politics of Menstruation*, why this is. She told me she believes that feminists have shied away from talking about menstruation because it sheds light on a major difference between male and female bodies, and feminism is about equality. If feminists acknowledge the fact that our bodies are different, Bobel says, "they're afraid it will be used against us."[15]

But that's the thing. Menstruation has always been used against women, and still is today, albeit more subtly.

The Curse: A Cultural History of Menstruation states, "In the U.S. today, outright cooking and segregation taboos are just a cultural memory. The emphasis is on behaving normally during the menstrual period ... today's woman is determined to prove that she can do her job 'like a man.'"

More than thirty years ago, the authors of *The Curse* recognized that Western society was not structured to serve the menstruating woman. The message from society is reinforced by advertising: we must conceal menstruation at all costs and act like it's not even happening. A favourite slogan of today's period positive posse is, "Anything you can do I can do bleeding." While certainly true, should we have to?

To be clear, I do believe that we *are* all equal and that we deserve equal rights regardless of our sex or gender identity. At the same time, I recognize that the packages we come in are different. While male hormones do cycle (on a twenty-four-hour cycle versus a monthly one), there is no equivalent to menstruation in the male body. There is no male counterpart to the uterus. These differences don't make one sex or gender superior to the other. Just different. And when you start to take a look around, you'll see that the world was built for one type of body — and that extends far beyond menstrual cycles and includes race, ability, age, body shape, and size.

While menstruation may not be at the forefront of modern feminism, activists have been focused on this issue for decades, long before periods went public in 2015. In 2010, Bobel's book chronicled the history of menstrual activism that had in fact started decades earlier on the fringes of feminism. It was the hard work of women throughout the sixties, seventies, eighties, and nineties that paved the way for those Instagram-worthy moments of 2015, and certainly my own podcast and book, to launch menstrual activism into the mainstream.

Born of the women's health movement of the sixties and seventies, menstrual activism really took shape during the toxic shock syndrome (TSS) crisis of the late seventies and early eighties. More than 1,200 cases of toxic shock were reported in the United States and Canada between 1976 and 1981, with at least three reported deaths in Canada alone.[16] Super-absorbent tampons made from rayon were linked to TSS. Feminist activists joined together with consumer advocates to work with the big four companies to ensure that products were safe. More than ten years later, in 1992, this work culminated in regulations that standardized tampon absorbencies and labelling.

In her book, Bobel sketches portraits of the two wings of menstrual activism: the radical, anti-establishment activists DIYing their own products in response to the TSS crisis, and the feminist spiritualists celebrating their own flow. The two movements, which I brushed up against as a young woman, certainly influenced my own flow and the trajectory of my life. While the punk rock menstrual activists were rejecting the big four menstrual brands, the feminist spiritualists were celebrating the "divine feminine" and the connection between nature and their menstrual cycles through new moon ceremonies and modern-day red tents.

TRADING THE TYRANNY OF SHAME FOR THE TYRANNY OF PERIOD POSITIVITY

So, did 2015 move the needle in terms of busting shame and taboo around periods?

While it may be too soon to call, one thing is certain: people are talking about periods in public like never before. Many of the events that put periods at the forefront in 2015 used shocking images to grab the public's attention. These tactics are designed to do just that — grab headlines, launching the issues related to period shame, stigma, and inequity into the mainstream conversation. These tactics are important, but as a movement, menstrual activism is about more than shock and awe.

Before we can talk about access to safe, reliable menstrual management products or education designed to provide true body literacy, we need to be able to talk about periods. In public. And not just within the context of complaining about adverse side effects or what you use to manage the blood.

"How to Break a Curse" is the aptly named conclusion to Elizabeth Kissling's book, *Capitalizing on the Curse* — an examination of how corporations have capitalized on centuries of menstrual shame and taboo to sell solutions to problems that aren't really problems at all. The title sums up not only the book, but the entire modern menstrual activist movement. The curse of menstrual shame and stigma can be broken, and we hold the power to do so in our own hands.

Kissling writes that *"menstruation will no longer be a curse only when women determine how they relate to their menstrual cycles on their own terms"* (emphasis mine). In our current culture, most of us relate to our menstrual cycle only through the products we use to manage it. It's only acceptable to discuss menstruation within the context of what we use to mop up the blood, or to complain about PMS or other adverse side effects. The number of products available on the market gives us the illusion of freedom. We can choose from pads or tampons, flexi-wings, applicators, scented or unscented products, but at the end of the day it's really just the same thing in a different package.

In recent years we have begun to see real innovation in terms of menstrual products, although many of these new and innovative items come at a premium. Those who can afford the upfront costs of reusable products can choose from eco-friendly menstrual cups or period underwear. Organic tampons can be delivered right to your door, timed to arrive with your period.

Cloth pads, the very things the menstrual hygiene industry emancipated us from, are regaining popularity as women demand products that are better for both our bodies and the environment.

Many of the companies behind these products — and certainly the mainstream, conventional brands have also been catching on to this — market them with a "period positive" message.

The term "period positive" was first used by comedian and activist Chella Quint in 2006. As a movement, #periodpositive is a way to "break the cycle of secrecy, fear and misinformation about menstruation that leads to negative consequences like period poverty."[17] Ironically, part of the #periodpositive campaign is to challenge the marketing of menstrual products and the very brands that have since co-opted the message of period positivity.

More and more brands, particularly those offering "alternatives" to drugstore pads and tampons, are forgoing shame to sell their products, and their messages are instead ones of empowerment — your period won't hold you back and it's nothing to be ashamed of either. These products promise a "better" period experience. As with their conventional counterparts, education is a key component of their marketing strategy. These companies often use inclusive language and images, recognizing those who menstruate outside of society's gender binaries; they deploy the very things that we've been taught to be ashamed of — period stains, cramps, etc. — in their marketing messages. They even show blood, while conventional companies continue to use blue liquid. Many modern menstrual companies also have a charitable component to their business operations, donating a portion of their profits or partnering with organizations providing menstrual products to those who need them, often in the global South. Along with period positivity, they can also check menstrual equity off the list of things they've accomplished.

As a consumer, I am the target market for these products, and this marketing appeals to me. This is, quite frankly, how menstrual products should be marketed. However, a deeper look at these marketing messages reveals that it's really just the same old shit in a different pile. Selling period positivity alongside products — even if they are safer, more eco-friendly, or innovative, as these products *should* be — isn't getting at the root of the issue. It's still forcing people to relate to their menstrual cycle through consumer products. Bobel describes it as "trading one tyranny for another."

"The commercial exploitation of menstruation is arguably the best thing that ever happened to women — also the worst," Kissling writes.

And she's right: all around the world, in every single country, including our own, we see the devastating effects that lack of access to appropriate menstrual products, clean water, and sanitation has on young girls and women. It keeps them out of school and home from work, which, in turn, keeps them in poverty. Education and appropriate menstrual products are essential to their future.

Gloria Steinem was right to suggest that menstrual products should be free.

THE NORMALIZATION OF PERIOD PAIN

But access to products isn't the only thing that keeps girls, women, trans men, and non-binary menstruators home from school or work. Getting your period is a painful experience for many, if not most of us.

While modern menstrual activists are working to ensure that there's a tampon in every bleeding vagina, calls for better understanding of the menstrual cycle as a vital sign, and of period pain and other menstrual cycle-related disorders, are noticeably absent from the conversation.

In the spring of 2018 I attended a panel event in Toronto called Menstruation's Moment, where panelists spent more than an hour talking about all sorts of topics related to periods — from access to products both at home in North America and in Africa, to the need for trans-inclusive language in product marketing. But not once was pain or the discomfort associated with menstruation mentioned or alluded to.

I later asked the event organizers if period pain was deliberately left off the agenda. They agreed that while this was an important topic, the intention of the panel was to address the most pressing issues in menstrual equity and they couldn't cover everything.[18]

I couldn't help but wonder why menstrual pain, given that the vast majority of menstruators suffer during each cycle, didn't qualify as one of the most pressing. Is it simply because we all just assume pain is part of the menstrual experience?

Long before my period made an appearance, I remember complaining about having "cramps" with my childhood bestie. I didn't have cramps, but this is a telling story: from a young age I associated menstruation with being grown up and assumed that it was something that was painful and uncomfortable.

Probably because for the majority of us who get periods, it is. While statistics vary on how many people actually suffer from dysmenorrhea (the medical term for painful menstruation), the numbers usually fall anywhere between 45 and 95 percent. That's a lot of people who are experiencing some type of pain, often debilitating enough to interfere with the course of their everyday lives.

To put it another way: anywhere from a quarter to about half of the world's population experiences pain about once a month. Over the course of a lifetime, that could amount to about three thousand days, or just over eight years, spent in pain and discomfort. Research has shown that dysmenorrhea is responsible for the majority of short-term school absences among adolescent girls, and some studies have suggested similar findings in the workplace, although this has been more difficult to test.[19] Because of menstrual shame and taboo, it's likely that most of us aren't calling in sick to work with menstrual cramps and instead will use another excuse like a headache or food poisoning.

If menstruation is a sign that the female body is inferior or faulty, then menstrual pain doubles down on that theory. Anywhere else in the body, pain is a sign that something is wrong, yet it's generally accepted that menstrual-related pain is "normal."

In her book *Closer: Notes from the Orgasmic Frontier of Female Sexuality*, author Sarah Barmak writes about the "dysfunction" of female sexuality. Replace "sexuality" with "menstruation" and this paragraph is still strikingly accurate:

"Something is off about this picture. Being dysfunctional is so common that it's the new normal. If women are as likely to have some kind of complaint as they are of being 'functional,' do we need to rewrite our definition of 'functional'? What if female sexuality is not the problem — what if our idea of 'normal' is the problem."

Despite their prevalence, menstrual pain and menstrual-related disorders don't seem to be a hot topic for research. They receive little funding or attention from the medical research community. Laura Payne, an assistant adjunct professor at the UCLA Pediatric Pain and Palliative Care Program, suggests that the pervasive nature of menstrual pain simply makes it uninteresting from a research perspective: "It's possible that because it seems so common, it may not [be seen to] warrant further investigation."[20]

Endometriosis, a disease that affects at least one in ten worldwide, has no cure or even a reliable way to diagnose it outside of invasive surgical procedures. But if you've ever wondered how this debilitating disease affects the sex lives of male partners of patients with endometriosis, you're in luck — a 2017 study from the University of Sydney examined just that.[21] This is a striking example of the ways that the medical industry privileges male experiences over women's.

As Elizabeth Yuko, a bioethicist and writer, wrote when she coined the term the "period paradox" in an essay from online magazine *The Establishment*, periods have long been used as proof of women's inferiority — so much so that the fact a woman menstruates can disqualify her from public office and a number of other jobs in the eyes of some. Yet periods are still not taken seriously.

Menstrual pain is often poorly treated, or even disregarded, by health professionals and pain researchers; it's simply been accepted that pain is to be expected as part of the menstrual experience.[22] Even those people who are experiencing pain don't take it seriously.

Abby Norman, author of *Ask Me About My Uterus: A Quest to Make Doctors Believe in Women's Pain*, sums it up: "Nobody takes women's pain seriously, not even women."[23]

A study published in the *British Medical Journal* in 2015 found that symptoms perceived to be related to the menstrual cycle were often under-reported. The menstrual taboo has normalized period pain to the point that we don't even think that our pain is worth mentioning to a doctor, or we believe that nothing can be done about it. Perhaps that's why it takes, on average, about two years for a person experiencing extremely painful menstruation to even broach the subject with their doctor.[24]

Even then, once you finally open up to your doctor about your symptoms, will you be taken seriously?

It's easy to laugh out loud at the picture I presented of early medicine's gender bias and blatant disregard of female bodies — their misunderstanding of the way the body works seems comical from the perspective of modern society and today's medical establishment. After all, we now know so much more about the human body, regardless of sex. Female test subjects now must be included in medical research and drug trials, although this wasn't a requirement until the 1990s. Hell, women can now be doctors, and in fact are graduating more often from North American medical schools than men. But despite all of this *progress*, medical gender bias — a difference in the standard of care and treatment that patients receive in a medical setting based on their gender — continues to thrive.

An online poll from *Prevention Magazine* in 2018 asked readers if they've ever had a doctor dismiss their symptoms because of their gender. The results were overwhelmingly yes — 92 percent at the time of writing.[25, 26] Anecdotal evidence has long suggested that women are more likely than men to be undertreated or inappropriately diagnosed, particularly when it comes to pain. And now data supports those allegations.

Women having a stroke or heart attack are more likely to be misdiagnosed in an emergency room setting than men are.[27] When a woman presents to the ER with acute abdominal pain, she waits an average of 65 minutes for pain medication. Men wait 49 minutes.[28] Women are more likely to be given sedatives for their pain and men to be given pain medication.[29]

It's no wonder that we hesitate to talk to health care professionals about period pain.

EARLY MENSTRUAL EXPERIENCES INFLUENCE LONG-TERM ATTITUDES

How we learned about menstruation and our first experiences with menstruation in adolescence may shape how we view our periods throughout our lives. A 2004 study exploring the relationship between early and current menstrual experiences found that study participants who had negative early experiences of menstruation reported more negative attitudes than women in the positive group did. Those who had positive early and current menstrual experiences reported more positive body image and better general health behaviours.[30]

Who we learn about menstruation from may also be a factor. One study found that girls who learned more about menstruation from male sources rated menstruation as more debilitating and negative than those who learned less from male sources.[31]

The curse of menstruation extends far beyond monthly cramps or headaches. It has deep roots embedded in almost every corner of modern culture, from education to medicine.

So how do we break the curse?

Activists and organizations working in the global south have identified that education is the key to destigmatizing menstruation and improving the lives of girls. In fact, if time or money is an issue, and they have to prioritize education or products, education always wins.

The same goes for us here in North America and the Western world.

Before we can define menstruation on our own terms, we need to fill in the gaps that our health class education may have missed — or blatantly ignored. While a vast majority of people now know what periods are before the onset of menarche, what we learn about the menstrual cycle is the bare minimum, and it's generally in the context of fertility.

Instead of celebrating the first period, positioning the menstrual cycle as a vital sign, and highlighting the positive aspects that are likely more meaningful to adolescents than fertility — such as stronger bones and muscles, increased athletic performance, and heightened creativity — the sex education conversation is generally focused solely on birth control.

BIRTH CONTROL AND THE MYTH OF THE "REGULATED PERIOD"

Hormonal birth control has become the gold standard for treatment of heavy, painful, or irregular periods. When a young person begins to experience long cycles that are perhaps unpredictable, or painful cramps before and during their periods — which is completely normal for the first few years of menstruation as the endocrine system matures — they are often prescribed birth control as a way to treat the pain and "regulate their periods."

A study by the Guttmacher Institute found that more than half of those on "the Pill" were using it for reasons other than contraception. Of that group, more than 80 percent of users between the ages of fifteen and nineteen were using it for non-contraceptive reasons such as menstrual pain or regulation.[32]

But here's the thing — birth control doesn't regulate your periods, and the period you experience while on the pill isn't actually a period at all. Birth control doesn't "make your body think it's pregnant," as is often the belief among users — it shuts down your menstrual cycle by replacing your body's natural hormones with synthetic ones.

The "period" that you experience when taking hormonal birth control is a withdrawal bleed. When you stop taking the hormones, it triggers a bleed — something that was added as a marketing technique in the early days of the pill to make it seem more natural to appease the Catholic Church.[33] When the pill was first introduced, women believed that having a regular menstrual cycle was a sign of good health and were hesitant to take a medication that would make their periods go away. I wonder where they might have got an idea like that, eh?

Every so often you'll see a headline espousing that doctors say you don't need to have your period while you're on the pill, which is true. Since you're not actually having a true period, there's not actually a real physiological reason for the bleed. But these articles rarely, if ever, discuss the differences between your menstrual cycle and why it's important, and what happens when you're taking hormonal contraception.

What we really should be investigating are the benefits of your menstrual cycle and the safety of suppressing the menstrual cycle for long periods of time.

Women of my mother's generation took birth control for a couple of years here and there between pregnancies without adverse effects on their health or fertility. But we are the first generation of women and girls to start using it in our teen years and well into our twenties and thirties, and beyond; birth control is now regularly prescribed to women in their forties experiencing irregular periods as a result of perimenopause. While we're often assured that the risks associated with hormonal birth control are low, we don't yet know what the long-term effects will be.

When you're not on hormonal birth control, your hormones fluctuate throughout your menstrual cycle. As estrogen rises in the first half of your cycle, it thickens the uterine lining. A surge of hormones triggers ovulation, and then your body starts to produce progesterone for about ten to fourteen days. If an egg hasn't been fertilized, progesterone dips and the uterine lining is shed — in other words, you get your period.

With hormonal contraception, the hormonal fluctuations are replaced with a steady stream of synthetic hormones — which hormones and how much will depend on the type of birth control being used. The uterine lining stays thin; this is why "periods" are often lighter and shorter while using hormonal birth control. And it's the withdrawal of synthetic hormones that creates a disruption in the uterine lining, causing it to bleed.

In *Take Control of Your Period — The Well-Timed Period: From Quality-of-Life to Cancer Prevention* — a book that's not really about taking control of your period but rather a two-hundred page advertisement for a brand of birth control introduced in 2003 that reduces the number of "periods" the user has to just four a year — the author, Diane Kroi, M.D., argues that having a monthly period doesn't offer any special health advantages; there is no known medical benefit to having a monthly period, even if you're not using synthetic hormones and have a "natural" cycle.

She isn't wrong. In my research, the only health benefit of menstruation I found was a slight possibility of the reduction in the risk of stroke as a result of lowered iron stores.[34]

But the argument that there are no health benefits to your period is simply missing the plot. Because your period isn't just your period — it's a part of your menstrual cycle, which *does have* numerous health benefits, and it's perhaps not even the most important part of it! Conventional Western medicine parses out the body into parts, treating each one individually with little thought to the big picture. As a holistic health practitioner who looks at the overall health picture, I find the idea that you can simply shut off a single bodily function without consequence to be extremely short-sighted.

The ability to choose when — or if — to have children has greatly benefitted the advancement of women around the world, thanks to hormonal birth control. I am one of them — I used hormonal birth control of one type or another for well over a decade, and I did not become pregnant when I didn't want to.

However, hormonal birth control is not without its risks — they are printed right there on the package. In general, these medications are safe and the side effects are rare or low risk. But what the pharmaceutical industry, mainstream medicine, and the news media has to say about hormonal birth control seems to contrast sharply with what is actually happening with the women who are taking it. The lived experience of taking hormonal birth control is very different from what is advertised on the package or communicated through the media.

It's not blood clots or increased blood pressure that many women are dealing with; in reality, it's more subtle, harder to put your finger on. It's a shift in your moods, simply just not *feeling like yourself*, something that I can certainly relate to.

For as long as I can remember, throughout my twenties, I always felt like something wasn't right in my life. I was working hard, going to school, getting great jobs and excelling at them. But there was always something that was *off* — not quite a feeling of dissatisfaction, but something felt missing, like I wasn't really living my truth. It was this feeling that eventually led me to leave my job as a successful public relations professional at a busy PR agency to study nutrition. By the time I came out the other side, graduating from nutrition school, everything in my life had changed. I had stopped taking hormonal birth control, and, for the first time in my life, I was cycling naturally. I then became pregnant. I had left the corporate world entirely and for the first time in my life I finally started to really feel like myself.

Could it have been that the hormones I took for all those years hadn't just suppressed my menstrual cycle, but also that part of me that I always felt was *just* out of my reach?

I found menstrual activism as a young teenager, as my interest in reproductive health and sex brushed up against my punk rock roots and introduced me to DIY pads. I loved making zines about toxic tampons and sewing my own pads. I became a sort of medicine woman among my friends; I was the one who could help you navigate a missed or late period, a yeast infection, or whatever other weird thing was going on in your underwear.

But after high school graduation, I felt the pressure to get a real job, to join the corporate world. I excelled in the corporate world because I was able to work almost constantly — save for the migraines I got once a month. I got in to the office early and stayed late. I had no work-life balance because there were no boundaries between the two. I was a fantastic worker.

When I launched the *Heavy Flow* podcast and began to dive deep into menstrual activism and the sister issues that come with it — the long-term use of hormonal birth control, fertility awareness, sex education — I started to wonder if maybe that part of me that felt missing all those years was because I was on the pill. If I hadn't been on it, would I have made the same decisions? Would I have succumbed to the capitalist work ethic that made me value only how productive I was in my life?

Of course, I'll never know — I can only speculate. And if I think too hard about these questions, it's almost too painful to consider. I really and truly felt grief for all the cycles that I never had, for all the missed opportunities that I had to connect with my body.

I know I'm not the only one. Join a birth control side-effect related group on Facebook and you'll find hundreds, if not thousands, of others who felt the same vague sense of *not being myself* while taking hormonal contraception.

HORMONAL CONTRACEPTION AND LONG-TERM FERTILITY

These young women who are taking the birth control pill in their teens as a way to control painful periods, heavy bleeding, or irregular cycles are often assured that their fertility will be preserved until the time comes that they want to have a baby. This is another area where there's a vast disparity between the official, biomedical party line and the actual lived experience of those who are taking hormonal contraceptives.

In 2009, a study of two thousand women looking at the rates of conception after stopping birth control concluded that 72 to 94 percent of women who had taken hormonal birth control were pregnant within one year of cessation; about the same as women who had been using non-hormonal methods such as condoms.[35] But just like the physical, emotional, and mental changes associated with being on hormonal contraception, what women are reporting seems to be a different story.

Many women struggle with conceiving after they have stopped taking hormonal contraceptives. While some women stop taking hormonal contraceptives and start ovulating right away, it's not the case for many, who may experience long periods of amenorrhea, or irregular or unpredictable periods, after stopping.

Many doctors say that it takes about eight months for ovulation to return after stopping hormonal contraceptives, but Lisa Hendrickson Jack, a holistic reproductive health practitioner who teaches Fertility Awareness Methods (FAM) for charting and interpreting your menstrual cycle, says that's simply not always true. She has worked with countless women who have struggled to regain their menstrual cycles and fertility after coming off hormonal contraception.

It's not eight months, but rather eight *cycles* that it takes for ovulation to return after stopping hormonal birth control.[36] That can be a drastically different time frame. If you experience a long period of amenorrhea following the pill and longer cycles, it might take a year or two before you've actually had *eight cycles*. It's a frustrating place to be in when trying to conceive.

Many young women are taught to treat their fertility like an enemy, fighting against it by shutting off their menstrual cycles in order to avoid pregnancy, unaware of the important health benefits of the menstrual cycle and the other options available to manage fertility. It's common that women are advised that when they want to get pregnant, they just have to stop the pill — but it seems that that's simply not always true.

We can't blame it all on hormonal contraceptives; there are, of course, other factors at play. For one, women are delaying pregnancy.[37]

Delaying pregnancy until later in life means the chances of conceiving during each cycle drop. In your twenties you have about a 30 percent chance of conceiving each cycle. By the time you're in your forties, the chances of conceiving after trying for a year is just 3 to 4 percent.

We have been conditioned to believe that getting pregnant is easy — we must take steps to avoid pregnancy at all times as you could become pregnant at any time during your cycle, hence the reason for birth control that's taken 365 days a year. In reality, the window of when you can actually conceive is small.

So, perhaps it's not hormonal birth control on its own that contributes to difficulty conceiving once you stop taking it, but the culture that we have built around birth control. Getting a prescription in your teens is like a rite of passage, regardless of whether or not you're sexually active. I started taking hormonal birth control before I became sexually active; it was only later that contraception became a convenient side effect of my "regular periods." Being a woman means taking your pill — certainly I know I felt sophisticated and grown-up carrying that little packet of pills around in my purse (these were the days just before everyone had a cell phone, so there was little else in my purse at the time).

Hormonal birth control is a complicated topic that is difficult to unpack, but one that we must discuss alongside the menstrual myths. Being critical of the pill and all the other various incarnations of hormonal contraception is often seen as "anti-feminist," or tied to right-wing, anti-abortion politics. In recent years there seems to have been a line drawn between those who use hormonal forms of contraception and those that use "natural" birth control, or "fertility awareness," particularly among health and wellness influencers on social media. The message from many of these influencers is those who choose hormonal forms of contraception are "bad" and those that go *au natural* are "good."

Looking at birth control in such a binary way erases the very real benefits of hormonal contraception. For one, it works. I took hormonal contraception for many years and didn't get pregnant when I didn't want to. And if hormonal contraception isn't for everyone, non-hormonal or barrier methods aren't either. Some people have partners who are uncooperative or abusive; others have very stressful schedules or just simply can't or won't risk the chance of pregnancy.

Hormonal birth control can also bring relief for those suffering from diseases that can be very painful, such as endometriosis, adenomyosis, and ovarian cysts, or from polycystic ovarian syndrome, which is often marked by very long, irregular cycles. In the absence of cures for these complex hormonal disorders, hormonal birth control, while imperfect, may be the best — or only — option.

The blanket statement that hormonal birth control is "bad" oversimplifies a complex topic and takes the focus away from the real debate we should be having, which is why aren't we creating long-acting, reversible birth control methods that don't destroy our hormonal ecosystem?[38]

The answer, of course, lies in the deep-rooted patriarchy that is inherent in our medical system and our views of the female body. Our societal attitudes around birth control are closely linked to our misunderstanding of menstrual cycles and our underestimation of its importance to our health and wellness beyond fertility. For as long as medical history has been documented, medicine has had a gross misunderstanding of the female body and how it works. Because, to put it in no uncertain terms, for centuries men have given zero shits about figuring out how the female body works and how it may be different from — *not just inferior to* — male bodies.

As a result, we have a much greater tolerance for what we feel is okay to do to a female body than we do for a male body. In clinical trials of male birth control pills, many men have dropped out of the trials because of side effects, including depression and lower libido. Sound familiar? Those are two well-documented side effects of female hormonal birth control pills that we have simply accepted as the norm. There is nothing shocking about a woman with a low libido. Even today, with all of our liberated sexual freedoms, the myth that women are simply "less sexual" than men continues to thrive. So, when a woman feels like her sex drive is low or her libido has all but disappeared when she's taking hormonal birth control, it's not considered a serious complaint because her sex drive is thought to be where it ought to be: non-existent.

Holly Grigg-Spall, author of *Sweetening the Pill: Or How We Got Hooked on Hormonal Birth Control*, argues that when it comes to hormonal birth control, we don't really have choice, just the illusion of it. Capitalism masquerades as choice because we can choose between the pill, the patch, the ring, the hormonal IUD, the implant, or the shot.

For those of us who have a choice when it comes to birth control, on what basis are we making those choices? The backbone of the midwifery model of care is informed choice — the idea that you can only truly decide what is right for you or your body when you understand the risks and benefits of all options presented to you.

If we don't understand how birth control acts on our bodies, and if we don't understand how our bodies even work, what kind of choices, about birth control and otherwise, are we really making?

♦ PART 1 ♦
THE BIOLOGY

CHAPTER 1
GETTING TO KNOW YOUR BODY

While it's likely that most of us who grew up in North America learned what menstruation was before we got our periods — if not from a formal reproductive health program at school, then certainly from television commercials, older siblings or friends, or perhaps our parents — we probably weren't taught much more than the basics. When you get your period, you'll bleed about once a month or every twenty-eight days; you'll need a pad or tampon to manage the blood; it's probably going to be, at best, uncomfortable; and last, but certainly not least, this means that now you can get pregnant.

Now that we understand the cultural forces that have been keeping us from understanding and claiming the power of our menstrual cycles, it's time to get to know our cycle and the power that lies within — the critical role that it plays in our health beyond fertility, the possibility of using our hormonal ebbs and flows to our advantage, and the connection between menstruation and something more.

The good news is that your menstrual cycle is yours. You don't need a doctor or any special equipment like a speculum or an ultrasound machine to really get to know and understand it. A mirror and a thermometer are helpful, but also completely optional! A little information can go a long way toward empowering and advocating for yourself.

Claiming your menstrual cycle goes beyond just understanding how it works — it's about body literacy, the ability to read and understand the signs and signals of your menstrual cycle and understanding *your* body within the context of what's normal. When you know yourself, you can use your menstrual cycle as a lighthouse that guides your overall health and wellness.

At the end of the day, my mission is to provide education to everyone on this planet who has a menstrual cycle. Only when you know what is happening to your body can you truly make informed decisions about what is right for you — that goes for choices around birth control methods, family planning, medical procedures, sex, medications, food, menstrual products — any decision that has an effect on your body.

The first step to claiming your menstrual cycle is to understand the physiology of your body. What exactly is happening every month? What body parts are involved? And how does this affect your day-to-day wellness?

Once you have a solid understanding of how your menstrual cycle works, you can observe your own cycle by tracking or charting it. This allows you to get to know what's happening with your body and to identify hormonal imbalances and adjust your nutrition or lifestyle. Your cycle will act as a guide to your overall health.

At its most basic, the physiological function of the menstrual cycle is to prepare your body for pregnancy, although fertility isn't the only reason why the menstrual cycle is valuable to your health and wellness. As we'll discuss in the following chapters, your menstrual cycle is a vital sign that's both an indication and promoter of your overall health and wellness.

Menstrual cycles are one of the things that set female bodies apart from male bodies; there is no functional or physiological equivalent in a male body. I want to differentiate that what I mean by this is sex, in a phenotypical body, and not gender, which is much more nuanced. I also want to acknowledge that periods aren't what make you a woman. There are plenty of people who identify as a woman who don't menstruate — for reasons such as menopause, medication, hormonal contraception, or health issues that suppress ovulation — and many people that don't identify as a woman who do.

Today, we in the West are living longer and having fewer babies, which means that we're having more periods than ever before. In earlier times women spent most of their time pregnant or nursing. Most of us can expect to reach menopause, when the menstrual cycle stops.

Living longer also means living longer post-menopause. The average life expectancy for females in Canada is eighty-four; in the United States it's eighty-one.[1] That means we're now living a quarter of our lives or more in menopause. Many of the diseases that females are at risk for later in life, like breast cancer, heart disease — the leading cause of death for women — and osteoporosis, are the very things that consistent ovulation protects against.

Those that argue that we don't really need periods sometimes blame "incessant menstruation" — having regular periods for the better part of our adult lives, about forty years — as a contributing factor for female health issues. Laura Wershler, a veteran sexual and reproductive health advocate, stresses that it is inconsistent ovulation that contributes to women's health issues, not incessant menstruation.[2] The importance of ovulation to bone, breast, brain, and heart health is not something that can be underestimated.

So, let's get down to basics, shall we? It's time to learn everything about our menstrual cycles that we *didn't* in high school health class.

REPRODUCTIVE ANATOMY AND GENITALS

Let's start this journey into discovering the magic of menstruation with a look at the female reproductive system and genitals. Sometimes our internal organs feel very far away, which contributes to things like menstruation and reproductive health feeling mysterious. But they're really not.

I don't blame you for being oblivious to what's literally hidden right under the surface — much of the education you may have received about menstruation as an adolescent had more to do with selling products than actually educating you about your body and giving you the tools to understand it. When I first started teaching workshops about menstruation, I assumed that people just knew what body parts were involved, until I got questions like "Can I pee with a menstrual cup in?" or "What exactly is a uterus anyway?" Don't be ashamed if you haven't gotten intimate with your parts — it's never too late to get to know your own body.

Understanding your anatomy is a critical component of body literacy. It helps to demystify reproductive health and menstruation by helping you situate these processes within your body. Knowing your anatomy is also useful when advocating for yourself at the doctor's office. Telling your doctor that you're experiencing pain in your vagina is the not the same as pain in your vulva.

We're going to consider both the internal reproductive anatomy and the external genitalia — what they look like, where they are, and what they do.

A disclaimer: bodies are amazing and incredibly unique, which means that there are any number of variations on what is "normal" in terms of the way that they look. Some variation in size and shape is not only perfectly normal, but to be expected. We are all beautiful, unique snowflakes.

So, if your body doesn't look exactly like what is pictured here, know that's totally okay — it's not that your body is wrong or bad, it's just that the limitations of this book are such that I was unable to include several dozen images to ensure that everyone is represented! And if your only exposure to vulvas other than your own is through pornography, you might be surprised to learn how different various vulvas can look. Check out the Labia Library online at www.labialibrary.org.au for a beautiful gallery of vulvas of all shapes, sizes, and colours!

DECOLONIZING THE FEMALE ANATOMY

Surprising to no one who has a female reproductive system, the road to modern gynecology was paved with misogyny, racism, and abuse (for example, experiments were often carried out on black female slaves against their will). Medicine is also steeped in patriarchy, and many body parts, reproductive or otherwise, are named after the men who "discovered" them. For example, fallopian tubes are named after Gabriel Fallopian. And Ernst Grafenberg is the one who "discovered" the infamous, elusive G-spot. Some feminist health practitioners and linguistics experts argue that continuing to use these names perpetuates medical gender bias, and body parts should instead be renamed with descriptors that are meaningful and useful to the body's owner. I have chosen to use descriptive terms as much as possible.

The Phenotypical Female Reproductive System
Ovaries
Ovaries are about the size and shape of an almond and contain up to a million immature eggs at the time of birth — as in *your* birth. Each egg is contained in an ovarian follicle, a sac-like structure similar in shape and function to your hair follicles. Ovaries produce steroid hormones including progesterone and estrogen during the reproductive years. Most of us have two, although it's possible for your reproductive system to function with just one!

Corpus Luteum
After ovulation, the ruptured follicle is transformed into the corpus luteum (see Figure 3), which produces progesterone and eventually degenerates, either at the end of the menstrual cycle or in early pregnancy when the placenta takes over progesterone production.

Oviduct/Ovarian Tubes (Fallopian Tubes)
These ducts receive the egg after ovulation and provide a site where fertilization can occur. Each tube is about ten centimetres long. Ducts are not directly connected to the ovary.

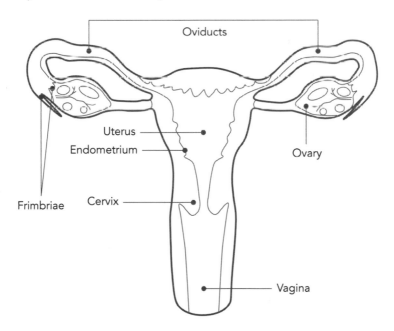

FIGURE 1 - PHENOTYPICAL FEMALE REPRODUCTIVE ANATOMY

Fimbriae

These finger-like projections create fluid currents that work to carry the egg into the uterine tube where it begins its journey to the uterus. Not all eggs make it to the uterine tubes, as the fimbriae often "miss" (despite having just one job).

Uterus

Put your hands under your belly button — there's your uterus, just under the surface. Some prefer to refer to it as the womb or womb-space. About the size of a lemon and the shape of an upside-down pear, it's a hollow organ that receives, retains, and nourishes a fertilized egg. Throughout your cycle, the uterine lining builds up and is either shed during menstruation or remains to nourish a pregnancy.

Cervix

A narrow opening that connects the uterus and vagina below. It acts as a physical barrier to protect the uterus from bacteria and infection. Looking at a diagram of the reproductive system, it's easy to assume your cervix is deep inside you, but it's really not — just about a finger's length away from the opening of your vagina.

The cervix opens and closes during ovulation and menstruation and dilates up to ten centimetres during childbirth. Throughout the menstrual cycle, the cervix hardens and softens and moves around within the vaginal canal. Glands in the cervix produce cervical mucus, the primary sign of fertility. This mucus helps to move sperm through the uterus to meet an egg in the oviducts, and even helps to eliminate sperm that may have genetic defects or are not strong enough to reach the uterine tubes. During pregnancy, the cervix creates its own mucus plug to seal the uterus.

Vagina

About eight to ten centimetres long, the vagina is an elastic, muscular passage between the vulva and the cervix. It creates a passage for menstrual blood to flow from the uterus, acts as the birth canal, and stretches during penetrative sex.

The Vulva and External Genitals

If you've been calling your external genitalia your vagina, then allow me to introduce you to your vulva. Your vulva is the external portion of your

TYPE BOOKS
THANKS FOR VISITING TYPE

9209 Reg 1 7:23 pm 27/02/19

S HEAVY FLOW	1 @	22.99	22.99
S TOUGH GUYS HAVE F	1 @	24.50	24.50
S GOOD EGG	1 @	21.99	21.99
SUBTOTAL			69.48
TAX: HST5 - 5%			3.47
TOTAL SALES TAX			3.47
TOTAL			72.95
DEBIT CARD PAYMENT			72.95

Ask about our programs and events!

Sorry no refunds. Exchange or
store credit within two weeks with
receipt. Thank you.

eans "sheath of
asize the penis
Sanskrit word
os."

gen
ant
bod
part

ris. It's an import-
ility to name your
cate for yourself,
nships.

Lab

The ... hich contains the

exte ... your vagina.

Grea

These glands (not pictured in Figure 2) flank the vagina and produce secretions to lubricate the outer end of the vagina when aroused.

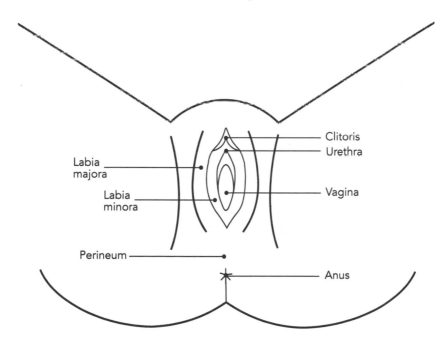

FIGURE 2 - PHENOTYPICAL EXTERNAL FEMALE GENITALIA

Clitoris

The outer part of the clitoris that is visible on the vulva is referred to as the glans and is covered by the clitoral hood. But this is quite literally the tip of the iceberg; the clitoris also has wings that reach out from the glans inside your body and down around the urethra and vaginal opening. The clitoris is made of sensitive erectile tissue that contains many nerve endings, becoming swollen with blood during arousal.

Labia Minora

The internal folds of the vulva, covering the vaginal opening.

Perineum

The space between the vagina and the anus.

Anus

The external opening to your colon.

Urethra

The tube that drains urine from the bladder.

HORMONES: THE BAND MEMBERS OF YOUR HORMONAL ORCHESTRA

Now that we've learned about where our parts are and what they do, let's look at the chemistry that makes them work. I'm talking about hormones.

"You're being hormonal!" is often used as an insult or a way to gaslight women into believing their lived experiences are all in their heads. However, hormones play a critical role in your body and how it functions. They are implicated in every single function your body performs from your heart beat to your stress response, appetites, energy levels, and pretty much every bodily function you can think of. These chemicals produced by your endocrine system — the second most important system in your body after the central nervous system[3] — carry messages between the cells and organs of your body.

There are about fifty hormones working away in your body at any given time, and they all work together. Think of your hormones as an orchestra — when even just one instrument is out of tune, it can throw off the whole band. The same goes for your hormones; if even just one is out of balance, it can affect your entire endocrine system and eventually lead to adverse health symptoms. Depending on which hormones are affected and why, symptoms can range from constipation to menstrual problems, from hair loss to issues regulating body temperature.

Your hormones are very sensitive to lifestyle factors such as nutrition, sleep, travel, illness, and in particular, stress. The good news is that works both ways — your nutrition and lifestyle can help your hormone function. But more on that later.

Menstrual Cycle Hormones

There are two types of hormones at play during your menstrual cycle: the hormones (progesterone and estrogen) produced by the ovaries; and those that are produced by your brain — the gonadotropin (GuRH), luteinizing (LH), and follicle-stimulating (FSH) hormones. Female bodies also produce and require small amounts of testosterone, the male sex hormone. Here's how they each work.

Estrogen

Probably the most familiar hormone, estradiol is one of three types of estrogen produced by your body, and it plays a key role in the menstrual cycle. Produced by follicles within your ovaries, the hormone's functions include thickening the uterine lining, producing cervical mucus, and maturing the egg released during ovulation. Estrogen isn't exclusive to your reproductive system; estrogen receptors are also found in cells in the vagina, bladder, breasts, skin, bones, arteries, heart, liver, and brain. An excess of — or "unopposed" — estrogen, not balanced by progesterone, can have many effects on menstruation, including heavy flow, long periods, and irregular cycles.

Follicle-Stimulating Hormone (FSH)

Produced by the pituitary gland, a major endocrine organ located at the base of your brain, follicle-stimulating hormone (FSH) does exactly what it says on the package: it stimulates the follicles within your ovaries to mature and release eggs during ovulation.

Luteinizing Hormone (LH)

Also produced by the pituitary gland, luteinizing hormone is responsible for both stimulating and completing follicular growth along with FSH.

Perhaps even more amazingly, LH is responsible for the luteinization of the ruptured follicle in order to transform it into the corpus luteum (a temporary endocrine structure in the ovaries involved in the production of hormones, primarily progesterone) following ovulation.

Gonadotropin-Releasing Hormone (GnRH)

GnRH is manufactured by the brain's hypothalamus and stimulates the release of the FSH and LH hormones — referred to together as the gonadotropin hormones.

Progesterone

Produced by the adrenal glands and corpus luteum immediately following ovulation, progesterone increases body temperatures and nourishes the uterine lining, and holds and nourishes a pregnancy. It's the "glue" that holds up the uterine lining in your luteal phase, the second half of your cycle, and throughout pregnancy.

But progesterone's super powers don't stop there. It's a key hormone, and not just for reproductive health. It also protects against breast cancer,[4] boosts thyroid hormones, lightens your period, reduces inflammation, builds bones[5] and muscles, promotes sleep, protects against heart disease,[6] and calms the nervous system, making it easier to cope with stress.

Testosterone

Yes, female bodies also have and need testosterone for well-being. Testosterone is required for our sex drives, energy levels, muscle tone, and more. Unlike the other hormones listed here, which fluctuate throughout your cycle, testosterone remains pretty constant. In the final phase of your cycle, right before your period, progesterone and estrogen both drop and testosterone is the primary hormone. A marker of polycystic ovarian syndrome (PCOS) is an elevated level of androgens, or male sex hormones, which contributes to irregular periods, acne, and facial hair growth, among other symptoms.

CHAPTER 2
UNDERSTANDING THE MENSTRUAL CYCLE

Your period — the time in your menstrual cycle when you are bleeding — gets all the press. In reality, however, it's just one part of a large and important cycle that plays a key role in your health and wellness.

Understanding the entire menstrual cycle, from the first day of your period to the last day of your cycle, is key to true body literacy and can be incredibly empowering. Not only will you know and understand what is happening to your body on any day of your cycle, but you'll be better able to identify when things might be out of balance and to make truly informed choices when it comes to contraception and other health issues.

When we are well, our periods show up regularly and without much fanfare. Bad periods — painful, heavy, irregular periods accompanied by severe PMS symptoms — aren't just part of the female experience: they're a signal that your hormonal health is out of tune. Other times, a "bad period" can be a sign that something is happening in another body system that has an effect on menstruation. For example, people with bleeding disorders often have very heavy menstrual bleeding; and thyroid issues are often reflected in your menstrual cycle.

Our hormonal health is incredibly sensitive to what we eat, how much and how well we sleep, and our stress levels, which isn't a surprise once you've learned that hormones are an important factor in every one of our bodily systems, from digestion to heart rate.

While there are certainly guidelines for what is considered to be normal or healthy when it comes to your menstrual cycle, the one thing that I always tell my clients is that it's important to know *your* normal.

THE PHASES OF THE MENSTRUAL CYCLE

Your menstrual cycle is made up of four phases: *menstruation*, the *follicular phase*, *ovulation*, and the *luteal phase*. You may be surprised to learn that there is actually a pretty wide window when it comes to what's normal in terms of length and flow. The average twenty-eight days that we often hear about is just that, an average — it's completely normal to have a shorter or longer cycle. What's most important is getting to know *your* normal.

Menstruation

- Typically lasts between two and seven days.
- Prostaglandins, hormone-like substances, trigger uterine contractions to shed the uterine lining that was built up during your previous cycle.
- Some light cramping and fatigue are normal during this phase.
- Hormones estrogen and progesterone both start out low.

Follicular Phase

- Known as the estrogenic phase because estrogen is the dominant hormone and starts to rise as you approach ovulation.

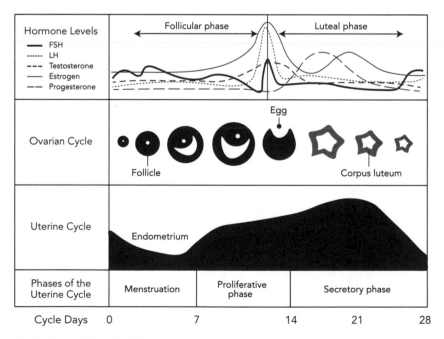

FIGURE 3 — THE MENSTRUAL CYCLE

- Estrogen steadily rises as your ovaries get ready to release the egg at ovulation.
- Lasts from seven to twenty-one days.
- Can vary in length from person to person, month to month; it's not unusual to have some variation of your follicular phase by a day or two each cycle.
- Very sensitive to stress and lifestyle.
- Uterine lining is building up.
- Cervical mucus changes from dry and sticky to slippery, "egg white" mucus.

Ovulation

- A surge in luteinizing hormone and follicle-stimulating hormone trigger the mature egg to be released from the follicle.
- Estrogen drops.
- Cervical mucus looks like "egg whites."
- Accounts for one day of the menstrual cycle.
- The ruptured follicle restructures into the corpus luteum, which begins to produce progesterone.
- Can sometimes cause pain known as mittelschmerz, or mid-pain — sharp, jabbing or burning sensation at the point of ovulation when the egg is released, or light bleeding.

Luteal Phase

- From the day of ovulation to the day before you get your period.
- Known as the progesterone phase.
- Estrogen has peaked before ovulation and is starting to fall.
- Progesterone now kicks in and is the dominant hormone.
- This phase is ten to sixteen days long and is finite. It might be shorter if there is a lack of progesterone, but it cannot be longer because the corpus luteum — the structure created from the follicle once an egg is released — can only survive for about two weeks.
- You will get your period about two weeks after ovulation.

- If no egg is implanted, progesterone and estrogen both drop, triggering the start of menstruation and a new cycle.
- In the few days before and during your period, estrogen and progesterone levels drop below testosterone levels.

A VITAL SIGN, NOT A CURSE

The menstrual cycle has everything to do with fertility — it is, after all part of our reproductive system and how we reproduce — yet it has so much more to do with your health and wellness than just your ability to make and have a baby.

Of all the menstrual myths out there, the idea that your menstrual cycle is only valuable if you're trying to get pregnant is perhaps the most far reaching — it's entwined with other issues around sexuality, birth control, and menstrual suppression. And it ignores emerging evidence that your menstrual cycle, and in particular ovulation, is both an indication and promoter of good health.

In 2015, the American College of Obstetricians and Gynecologists (ACOG) issued a statement that the menstrual cycle should be considered a vital sign in adolescents.[1] But even before the ACOG's statement, the Society for Menstrual Cycle Research (SMCR), a collection of interdisciplinary researchers, scholars, and activists, had been pushing for recognition of the menstrual cycle as a vital sign — not just for adolescents, but for anyone with a uterus of any age, from menarche to menopause.

In New York in 2004, more than a decade before the ACOG issued their statement, advocates for sexual and reproductive health met at a conference titled "The Menstrual Cycle as a Vital Sign." There, Paula Hillard, M.D., professor of obstetrics and gynecology and pediatrics at the University of Cincinnati College of Medicine, stated, "The menstrual cycle is a window into the general health and well-being of women, not just a reproductive event."[2]

> Your period is not just your period. It is an expression of your underlying health. When you are healthy, your menstrual cycle will arrive smoothly, regularly, and without undesirable symptoms. When you are unhealthy in some way, your cycle will tell the story.
> — Dr. Lara Briden, *Period Repair Manual*

In other words, if you aren't menstruating, that is a sign that something else is going on with the body.

The fact that experts are calling for the menstrual cycle to be recognized as a *vital sign* is significant. Vital signs are clinical measurements used to measure your health or a physical condition.[3]

As a vital sign, your menstrual cycle can tell you about your health and wellness just like your blood pressure, heart rate, or pulse can. Hormonal imbalances, nutrient deficiencies, immunological issues, allergies, and other health issues can be expressed in the menstrual cycle, but you have to pay attention to your cycle in order to see and understand them.

It's not just your period that is a sign of good health, but the entire menstrual cycle. This point is often overlooked when it comes to health education and even within our own bodies. Your menstrual cycle is more than just menstruation — that's just a small part of it, and perhaps not even the most interesting or important part. This might come as a surprise given how much focus and weight is put on menstruation itself: periods get all the press (even if it's not the most positive coverage!).

Your period may be a small part of the menstrual cycle, but it's likely the most troublesome — many, if not most, menstruators experience at least some adverse side effects before or during their periods, whether it's cramping, headaches, mood swings, or digestive issues.

Studies vary and so it's hard to get a good handle on exactly how many people suffer from PMS, painful periods (known as dysmenorrhea), or other ill effects related to menstruation, but statistics range anywhere from 45 to 95 percent, depending on the study. In other words, most of us who get our period feel shitty when we do.

But don't confuse what's common with what's normal.

Your period doesn't exist in isolation; it's part of your larger menstrual cycle, a complex orchestra of hormones that fluctuate throughout the month, ebbing and flowing and affecting more than just your sex drive and your period. To use our menstrual cycle as a vital sign is to use it as a barometer of our overall health and wellness. When something is out of whack with our menstrual cycle, or we are experiencing a lot of pain or other symptoms as a result of our periods, it's a sign that there is a larger imbalance happening in the body.

The hormones that are responsible for your menstrual cycle are responsible for much more than just your monthly cramps and cravings. They have a critical role to play in other parts of your body outside of your reproductive system. In particular, progesterone, the crucial hormone of your menstrual cycle released following ovulation, has a number of important benefits beyond holding up the uterine lining in the luteal phase or during pregnancy. This hormone is essential, not only for your menstrual health, but also for bone, breast, brain, and heart health, among others. This supports the idea that the menstrual cycle, and ovulation in particular, is a critical factor in female health.

Let's take a look.

Bone and Muscle Health

Progesterone plays a role in bone mineral density, protecting against osteoporosis, a disease characterized by low bone mass and deterioration of bone tissue, which can lead to increased risk of fracture.[4] It also stimulates the growth of new muscle.[5]

Breast Health and Development

Both estrogen and progesterone play a role in breast development in adolescence. Breasts reach full maturity about a year after the first period, when the body is producing progesterone via ovulation. Normal to high levels of estrogen that aren't counterbalanced by progesterone, produced through regular ovulation, appear to be a risk factor for breast cancer and progesterone may be a treatment option for breast cancer in the future.[6] Progesterone is also needed to help to protect against breast tenderness in the PMS window.[7]

Nervous System

Progesterone has a number of benefits for your nervous system, and in particular for brain health. It acts as a "neurosteroid," helping the brain to recover from injury and contributing to brain development in utero. Progesterone helps you sleep and even helps to improve your mood. Sounds like a few good reasons to ovulate, if you ask me!

Heart Health

More women die from heart disease than any other condition — in part because early studies of heart disease and its treatment only included males; this is a problem because heart disease presents very differently in women.

In a large study of women with heart disease, researchers found that those with heart disease had lower levels of progesterone compared to those who didn't have heart disease. The findings also suggested that older women with heart disease are more likely to have had lower progesterone levels and anovulatory cycles in premenopause.

Another study found that monkeys with regular ovulatory cycles had little to no blood vessel disease, which leads to heart attacks, compared with those that had lower progesterone levels.[8]

Other Health Benefits of Hormones

Progesterone isn't the only hormone that plays a key role in health. Estrogen is perhaps the most well-known of all hormones, but it does have some negative connotations. Given that it is the primary female sex hormone, it's often given credit for women being "hormonal" as a way to explain behaviour that seems to run contrary to our ideal version of femininity.

Putting that BS aside, estrogen is also essential for health. Every single cell in our body is equipped with an estrogen receptor, which means we likely couldn't function without this vital hormone — or at least not very well. So, we have estrogen to thank for a lot more than just making us "hormonal."

Hormones work together like a well-orchestrated team. They need to be in balance in order to function, and, like stacked dominos, when one is knocked out of balance, it can topple the entire set.

Many of the diseases that progesterone protects against are diseases that we are most at risk for after menopause. Hence menstrual cycles, and ovulation in particular, are of particular importance, not just to our current wellness, but also to our future health.

I know that it's difficult to imagine taking care of yourself now for an abstract date in the future. As a nutrition student I always struggled with the lessons that touted longevity — I've always been wary of putting too much focus and attention on the future. Because I want to live my best life *today*, I don't want to have to wait to reap the benefits of good health.

But consistent ovulation doesn't just set us up for good health once we're past menopause. It's beneficial to our health at all stages of life.

Our bodies are elegantly designed and smarter than we give them credit for. Our stress response, for example, was designed to keep us safe from predators and other dangers during prehistoric times. Because of the fight-or-flight nature of the stress response, we're either going to run away from the source of the threat, or to stick around and fight it. The stress response is orchestrated by hormones. Cortisol, the main hormone of your stress response, is made by the same endocrine glands as progesterone, the main hormone of our menstrual cycles, which explains why stress has such an incredible influence on our menstrual cycles and fertility.

While infertility is a complex issue and beyond the scope of this book, there is a good reason why stress, in particular, shuts down ovulation. We need to ovulate in order to reproduce, and the body isn't going to reproduce if it senses that you're not in a safe position to carry a pregnancy. It's the same reason why amenorrhea is often associated with eating disorders, or even simply undereating (or not getting enough nutrition from the food that you are eating). If your body senses a famine, that there's not enough food to sustain a pregnancy and eventually a child, it's going to shut down the reproductive function. It knows that it's not a good time for you to get pregnant.

This response that our bodies have to stress has larger implications. Today's chronically stressed, overstimulated culture isn't good for our health. We know that stress is a factor in diseases such as heart disease and stroke, but it can also show up in our menstrual cycles. Our hormonal processes can be interrupted and thrown out of balance because of the high-stress lives many of us live.

When we use the menstrual cycle as a vital sign, we are able to detect the early signs and symptoms of disease.

Many of the most common complaints related to menstruation can be linked to an imbalance between estrogen and progesterone, two of the hormones key to our menstrual cycles. These hormones must be in balance in order for our menstrual cycles, and the rest of our bodies, to run efficiently and to promote and maintain our health.

When your menstrual cycle is only valued within the context of fertility, you may believe you don't need to worry about it until you're ready to have a baby (if at all). This only perpetuates another myth: that you can simply use hormonal birth control for a decade or more until you're ready to get pregnant. While the medical establishment maintains that birth control is safe and effective to use until you're ready to get pregnant, the actual experience of many people who take them is very different, and a large number of women struggle with cycle regularity after long-term use of hormonal birth control.

This idea also implies that once you're finished having babies — if you choose to have a baby at all — your period is just something to wait out until menopause, which again ignores the long-term health benefits of ovulation, both on your premenopausal and postmenopausal health.

WHAT DOES A NORMAL CYCLE LOOK LIKE?

Now that we understand the big picture, what our menstrual cycle is and why it's important, you're likely wondering what's "normal" when it comes to your period. Just like anatomy and the overall length of the menstrual cycle, periods vary from person to person, month to month, but there are some parameters that constitute a normal menstrual cycle and period.

Length

Your menstrual cycle should be between twenty-one and thirty-five days, although it's normal for cycles to be longer in adolescence and perimenopause. Within the context of a twenty-one to thirty-five-day menstrual cycle, your period bleed should last between two and seven days. The first day of your period is the first day that you have a steady, consistent flow — generally the first day that you reach for a product to manage your flow. This is day one of a new cycle. If you have light bleeding or spotting in the days leading up to your period, that counts as part of the luteal phase of your previous cycle. For example, three days of spotting and four days of steady bleeding doesn't make up a seven-day period. The spotting would be counted in your previous cycle and your period would just be four days.

Colour and Consistency

Generally, your period should be deep red, like the colour of cranberry juice, and free of large clots. Some clots are normal, particularly on the first day or two of your cycle when the lining starts to shed faster than your body can produce the anticoagulants needed to prevent the entire uterine lining from shedding all at once. That would be inefficient and also terrifying to experience. However, clots that are larger than about a quarter are red flags that shouldn't be ignored, as their presence can signal a serious issue beyond just hormonal imbalance. Most importantly, watch out for changes. If you've never experienced clotting and suddenly you are noticing large clots, you'll want to see your doctor or medical professional to find out what's changed.

It's normal for the colour of your menstrual flow to change over the course of your period. It might start off brownish, particularly if you have spotting leading up to your period, and then get brighter as your period progresses. This change is because of the age of the blood and whether it's been exposed to oxygen, which changes the blood's colour. Think about a used Band-Aid — the blood is bright red when you're first injured, but when you're ready to change the Band-Aid, the stain is dark brown.

While many health practitioners, including alternative and paramedical practitioners like naturopathic doctors, aren't too concerned with the specific colour of your menstrual blood, it is of great importance in Traditional Chinese Medicine. Traditional Chinese Medicine practitioners use the colour of menstrual blood to identify deficiencies or imbalances of qi (energy), liver, or kidney function.

Flow

Menstrual flow should be a maximum of about 80 mL over the entire course of your period — that's about sixteen soaked tampons, or two-and-a-half filled menstrual cups (note that the volume of menstrual cups can vary depending on the brand, size, and shape).

PMS and Pain

While some light cramping and fatigue is normal, premenstrual symptoms (PMS) or pain that interrupt your daily routine are not. PMS includes about 150 different symptoms, ranging from bloating, irritability, headaches, and back pain, to anxiety, depression, sleep problems, and a host of other physiological and psychological symptoms. Technically, symptoms of PMS should go away when your period starts, but in reality, many women continue to experience discomfort throughout their period. Cramps and other pains related to menstruation, known as dysmenorrhea, are common but definitely not normal.

If you have an underlying health condition, even if it's not an endocrine disorder or related to hormones, it may be exacerbated during your PMS window. Mental health issues like depression or obsessive-compulsive disorder (OCD) can flare up in the week or so before your period, as can asthma or skin conditions like eczema or psoriasis.

WHAT IS SPOTTING?

Any bleeding that occurs outside of your normal menstrual period is called "spotting." There are a number of reasons why you might be spotting including ovulation, hormonal birth control, or pregnancy. Bleeding outside of menstruation can also be a symptom of fibroids, cervical polyps or lesions, or an infection like pelvic inflammatory disease (PID). Consistently spotting in the days leading up to your period may be an indication of a hormonal imbalance, particularly low progesterone. Be sure to track any spotting and speak to your health care provider about it to rule out any serious issues.

KNOW YOUR FLOW

If you have a vagina, there are going to be times during your cycle when fluid is going to come out of it: your menstrual blood and your cervical mucus, what Nora Pope, a naturopathic doctor specializing in hormonal health, refers to red and white flow, respectively. What are these mysterious substances? How do you know if your cervical mucus is normal or needs to be checked out? And why does menstrual blood look and smell different from other blood?

Read on and get to know your flows.

Cervical Mucus

Produced by your cervix, cervical mucus changes in relation to the rise of estrogen in your follicular phase and has a distinct pattern throughout your cycle. While there are many variations of what's normal for your cervical mucus, in general it will go from dry to wet as you approach ovulation. At its most fertile it often resembles egg whites; it's clear and stretchy, although it's normal for it to be streaked with red or pink if you experience ovulation bleeding. The Beautiful Cervix Project is a great online resource for getting to know what cervical mucus looks like throughout your cycle.

Cervical mucus is an important signal of fertility. It's necessary for sperm nourishment and mobility, creates an alkaline medium to protect sperm from the acidic PH of the vagina, acts as a filtering mechanism, and helps sperm to move.

Cervical mucus isn't generally part of basic sex or reproductive health education — or is it? The Always Changing® campaign does make reference to "vaginal discharge," saying that it's perfectly normal. It doesn't, however, explain what it is or why it's an important part of your menstrual cycle. The fact that it's referred to as "discharge" and not what it is — cervical mucus, a sign of fertility and therefore health — gives it a negative connotation. Have no fear, they tell consumers; there is a solution that you can purchase in order to cope with this perfectly normal part of life — a panty liner, worn between periods to protect your underwear.

"Vaginal discharge" is another example of something that is perfectly normal that the feminine hygiene industry has labelled as a problem so that they can conveniently sell you the solution.

Of course, there are times that vaginal discharge *is* a sign of an infection or problem — if it's green, greyish, or brown; has an unpleasant odour or if it is accompanied by burning, itching, or any other discomfort, you're going to want to get it checked out. But most of the time it's normal and perfectly healthy — and if ovulation is an indicator of good health, so too is the appearance of cervical mucus. Perhaps if we learned more about what's normal for our cervical mucus we'd better be able to identify when we should be concerned.

When I learned to chart my cycles and came to understand how to read cervical mucus, a lightbulb went off over my head when I remembered an exchange I had had with my doctor several years earlier. At my yearly physical, I mentioned that I often noticed a clear, stretchy mucus in my underwear. She assured me that it was nothing to worry about and totally normal, that sometimes your vagina could get a cold and get runny just like your nose does. Only once I learned about cervical mucus and the role it plays in fertility did I realize that what I had been concerned about was probably healthy cervical mucus, not a cold!

Menstrual Blood

Despite its name and, at times, striking crimson colour, there's more to menstrual blood than just blood. It also contains mucus, vaginal secretions, and endometrial tissue that's been sloughed off the uterus.

It can vary in colour from bright pink to deep ruby red to dark brown, depending on hormone levels, the length of your cycle, and what day of your period you're on. The first day of your period is usually darkest, and any spotting that you may have had leading up to your new cycle can often be dark brown because it's older blood that's been hanging around for a while.

As you progress through your period, it will often change to look more like "fresh" blood.

Because it's not just blood but also tissue, menstrual blood has a different consistency than the blood found in your veins. If you have clots in your menstrual flow, this is the tissue that forms the lining of the uterus.

This tissue is also what gives menstrual blood an odour. When it first comes out, menstrual blood doesn't smell any different than the rest of your blood — it might have a slight coppery smell, but that's about it. However, as the tissue mixes with oxygen and bacteria and starts to break down, it may take on a slight odour. Many menstrual products include "odour protection" in the form of perfumes or fragrance. These products aren't doing anything to eliminate the odour; they're just covering them up and may not be doing you any favours. I recommend avoiding scented products, as the chemicals contained in them may be endocrine disrupting, meaning that they can mess with your hormones; they can also be irritating and inflammatory, with the potential for contributing to menstrual pain, imbalanced hormones, and other issues. Because tampons absorb menstrual blood internally, the blood hasn't yet had a chance to mix with the air in the same way that it does on a pad, making scented tampons a moot point.

If you're concerned about menstrual odour, first consider this: has there ever been a time when you've been able to smell somebody else's menstrual blood? I can't think of a single time when I've ever noticed the odour of menstrual blood on somebody else. I also challenge you to consider unpacking why it is that you think the odour of a perfectly natural, healthy, important bodily process is so gross.

Of course if you notice a stark change in the way your menstrual blood smells, particularly if it smells foul or fishy, you're going to want to get that checked out.

Finally, if odour is still something that you really can't get over, simply make sure that you're changing your pad frequently or try using a product that is worn internally like a tampon or menstrual cup.

YOUR CYCLE ON HORMONAL BIRTH CONTROL

When you take any form of hormonal contraceptives, the natural ebb and flow of hormones produced by your endocrine system is replaced with a flat line of synthetic hormones. In other words, your menstrual cycle is suppressed. The period that you experience while taking hormonal contraception isn't a period at all, but rather a bleed that is triggered by the withdrawal of the synthetic hormones. The parameters outlined above for what is normal apply to those who have a menstrual cycle and aren't taking hormone drugs. What's normal in terms of hormonal fluctuations and withdrawal bleeds depends on the type of contraception you're taking and the cocktail of hormones that it contains.

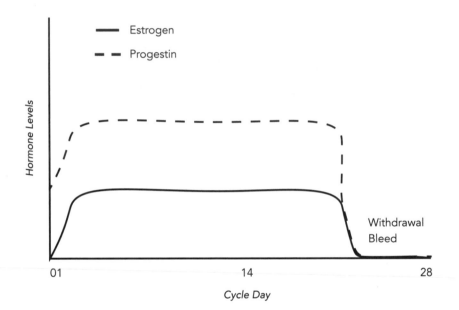

FIGURE 4 – AN EXAMPLE OF HORMONE LEVELS ON HORMONAL CONTRACEPTION

YOUR MENSTRUAL CYCLE AND YOUR LIFE CYCLE

When it comes to your period and menstrual cycle, what's normal can vary widely, depending on your age and whether or not you have been pregnant. It's not uncommon for the period that you had in your teen years to be different from the period that you have in your twenties or after childbirth.

The Centre for Menstrual Cycle and Ovulation Research (CeMCOR) defines four life phases that shape what our reproductive and menstrual health look like. They include the following:

1. Adolescence: From menarche, your first period, until about age twenty. Menstruation can begin between ten and fifteen years old, with the average age being twelve-and-a-half.
2. Premenopause: Age twenty until perimenopause.
3. Perimenopause: The time before and one year after the final flow. It can start any time between thirty-five and fifty-nine, with the average age forty-seven, and can last anywhere from five to fifteen years.
4. Menopause: Begins one year after the last flow.

When we start our periods, and throughout your teen years, it's completely normal for them to be far apart and unpredictable as the endocrine system matures. Cycles are often anovulatory, meaning the body is not actually ovulating despite having periods, and there may be a short luteal phase. Many teenagers experience cramps, heavy flow, irregular cycles, elevated levels of male sex hormones, and skin eruptions during this time — the very symptoms that often lead to patients being diagnosed with conditions such as PCOS and prescribed hormonal contraceptive therapy.

By our twenties, cycles should become more regulated and cramps often become less severe. Throughout this life phase, your menstrual cycles should be regular, and periods should appear with little to no discomfort.

IUDS AND YOUR PERIOD

Intrauterine devices, or IUDs, are small, T-shaped pieces of plastic, inserted into the uterus to prevent pregnancy by inhibiting sperm mobility and fertilization. There are two types of IUDs: hormonal, which use synthetic hormones similar to those found in other hormonal contraceptives, and non-hormonal, which uses a small amount of copper. IUDs have a higher rate of satisfaction than any other type of birth control and are highly effective, all without suppressing ovulation.

Either type of IUD can have an effect on your period. While hormonal IUDs can make your menstrual flow lighter, non-hormonal copper IUDs can have the opposite effect — it's not uncommon to have a heavier or "flooding" period along with severe cramps.

Other period-related side effects of the IUD may include irregular periods and mid-cycle spotting.

YOUR PERIOD AFTER PREGNANCY RELEASE

When to expect your period to return after childbirth is a common and lively discussion among new parents; yet just when you'll get your period, and what it will be like after you've had an abortion or miscarriage, is a topic that seems to still be shrouded in mystery. It comes with a double dose of shame and taboo when you combine menstruation with pregnancy loss or abortion.

While childbirth, abortion, and miscarriage are all very different experiences on the surface, they do share many similarities when it comes to how our bodies react. Samantha Zipporah, a holistic sexual health educator, activist, and advocate, describes this as the "universality of the womb continuum." To highlight the similarities, she reframes childbirth, miscarriage, and termination of a pregnancy as "pregnancy release." While the outcomes might be different, in all situations you were pregnant and then you were not. With that in mind, what to expect from your next period shouldn't be such a mystery.

Depending on when the pregnancy was released, you may experience a period of bleeding immediately after — this is referred to as *lochia* after childbirth — followed by a period of amenorrhea; or your cycle may return directly after.

If you experienced trauma as part of your pregnancy release — particularly around a miscarriage or traumatic birth experience — getting your period back may trigger a reaction to that trauma in the months or years following. If you have experienced trauma related to menstruation or find menstruation to be a triggering experience for you, I encourage you to seek appropriate mental health support, such as therapy. Some people find that using products worn internally such as a menstrual cup or tampon can help to keep the blood out of sight and avoid being triggered.

When Will My Period Return After Pregnancy?

When I was a new parent, I spent a lot of time in Facebook mom groups, and not a week would go by without at least one person polling the group to find out when their periods returned after baby. Those who enjoyed a year or more period-free were always met with jealousy, while condolences were offered for those whose cycles began soon after childbirth.

If I could tell you exactly when your period would return after pregnancy, I would be a very rich woman — it truly is a million-dollar question. The answer is, it depends, and science doesn't know exactly what it depends on.

Breastfeeding may delay the return of your cycle, as prolactin — a hormone produced when you are breastfeeding — indirectly suppresses ovulation. This is known as lactation amenorrhea. Many new moms get their cycles back around six to eight months postpartum, usually once the baby is starting to eat solid foods and breastfeeding less. But it's not uncommon for menstrual cycles to restart before that milestone, or well after. That said, breastfeeding isn't a guarantee that you won't be ovulating — that depends on how often the baby is feeding, if you're supplementing with formula, and your hormone and stress levels.

Dr. Claudia Valeggia, a biological anthropologist at Yale University, observed that lactation isn't the primary factor that determines when ovulation will begin again, but the availability of maternal energy. A study that looked at when menstruation began postpartum among the Toba women of Argentina found that two to three months of sustained weight gain was observed before menstruation, and therefore ovulation, resumed. This suggests that the brain has a monitoring system to detect when a woman has enough calories to sustain breastfeeding and the resumption of ovulation, which could lead to another pregnancy.[9]

The most important thing to know about your postnatal periods is that you're going to ovulate before your period shows up — which means that it's possible to become pregnant before you get your period back, so plan your contraception accordingly if you're not interested in becoming pregnant again! When you're breastfeeding, your cervical mucus may not go through the same changes from dry to egg white, as your hormone chemistry differs from when you're not breastfeeding. Toni Weschler, author of *Taking Charge of Your Fertility*, recommends watching for *any* changes to your mucus and considering that a sign of fertility.

If your pregnancy was released via abortion or miscarriage, the timing of your period's return can vary depending on how advanced the pregnancy was when it ended. Some women get their cycles back almost immediately, while others have a longer period of amenorrhea. Either way, remember that you will ovulate before you get your period, so if you're trying to avoid pregnancy ensure that you are using a form of birth control.

Why Is My Period Different After Pregnancy?

I hear from many clients, podcast listeners, and workshop attendees that their periods are different after pregnancy — while some seem to experience easier, lighter periods than before, the story I hear is often the opposite.

Pregnancy is a contributing factor to a heavy flow, although cramps may be reduced after pregnancy release. If you had a long period of amenorrhea postpartum, your first periods after your cycle returns might be heavier and come with more premenstrual symptoms as your body readjusts. Just like when you were a teenager and your period was a bit all over the place, your body will have a period of adjustment between pregnancy and the return of your regular menstrual cycle.

Why your period can be heavier after childbirth isn't quite clear. Heavier periods might simply be a case of physics — your uterus may be slightly larger or have a slightly different shape after childbirth, so there is more surface area to cover with the endometrium, which would mean more lining to be shed (what other part of your body went back exactly the same postpartum?).

If you were taking hormonal contraception before you were pregnant, which can shorten your period and lighten your flow, this may be the first time that you're experiencing "natural" cycles, so your postpartum periods may be more reflective of your body's natural state. Others switch from hormonal contraceptives to a copper IUD while breastfeeding, which can contribute to heavy or "flooding" periods.

If you're concerned about the length of time your period has been absent or changes in your period postpartum, talk to your primary health care provider and request a hormone panel to get a complete picture of your hormones.

Regardless of whether or not you're breastfeeding, life with a newborn or young child can be a time of high stress, little sleep, and less-than-optimal nutritional choices, which can wreak havoc on our hormones. I know what life with a small person is like. There's no shame in the eating-the-toddler's-leftovers-at-the-sink game, but it's also not the best thing for menstrual or hormonal health, and probably not for our happiness either. Supporting your hormones using the nutritional and lifestyle advice in the following chapter will help to promote ovulation and rebalance your hormones to manage symptoms like heavy flow and PMS, which may be worse after pregnancy.

IS IT PERIMENOPAUSE?

"Am I perimenopausal?" is one of the questions I'm asked most frequently. If we're not taught much about menstrual cycles, we're taught even less about menopause, a natural life event that is often looked at and treated as an illness rather than a normal life transition — even one that perhaps should be celebrated.

First of all, let's clear up some semantics. "Menopausal" is the state following your last period, so as long as you're getting your period, you're definitely not "menopausal" — not that there's anything wrong with that. It's possible that if you're starting to notice changes in your flow and/ or your hormonal health, you may be entering the very early phases of perimenopause, even if your cycles continue to be regular and normal in length. CeMCOR defines the onset of perimenopause as when a woman who is thirty-five or over starts to experience at least three of the following symptoms, either for the first time or with increased regularity or intensity:

- Heavier or longer menstrual flow
- Menstrual cycles shorten to less than twenty-five days
- Breast pain, swelling or lumpy breasts
- Menstrual cramps
- Mid-sleep wakening
- Onset of night sweats, especially before your period
- Migraines
- Premenstrual mood swings
- Weight gain without changes in exercise or food

Hormone levels change at the onset of perimenopause. While it was once thought that estrogen levels dropped during perimenopause, we now know that estrogen levels actually become higher, more variable and unpredictable, while ovulation becomes less frequent and progesterone levels are lower. It's this estrogen, unopposed by progesterone, that contributes to many of the symptoms that are often experienced during the perimenopause transition.

By the time you're thirty, hormone production starts to slow down and continues to decline throughout perimenopause until menstruation stops altogether: this is menopause. Some women may start to experience symptoms of very early perimenopause as early as thirty-five years old, even if their periods continue to be regular.

Perimenopause can last up to ten years or longer and varies widely from person to person. In a study of 344 women, researchers identified hundreds of variations of normal perimenopause.

During this time, you may experience changes in your flow including very heavy or "flooding" periods — you may be aware of what some call the "forties floods," irregular periods, fertility changes, sleep disturbances, cramping, night sweats, headaches, and more. Up to 80 percent of women experience hot flashes and/or night sweats, particularly around the beginning of their periods. When you're in perimenopause, night sweats can be sign that your period is about to begin.[10]

Periods become irregular and eventually stop. Menopause is official one year after the last period.

WHAT IF YOU FALL OUTSIDE OF NORMAL?

As you can see, there's a pretty wide range for what's considered "normal" when it comes to the length of your menstrual cycle and your period, depending on your age, whether or not you've been pregnant, and many other factors. That's why I encourage you to get to know what's normal for *you*, within the context of your current season of life.

While it's normal for there to be some variation in your cycle from month to month — a day or two here and there — if you are experiencing wildly different cycles each month, that can be an indication that your hormones are imbalanced.

If your menstrual cycle or periods fall outside of the parameters for what's normal, no matter what phase of life you might be in, it's not a reflection of you as a person. You haven't failed in some way or done something wrong.

Learning to look at your menstrual cycle as a vital sign means identifying potential imbalances and course-correcting by making dietary and lifestyle changes outlined in the following chapters to improve your menstrual and hormonal health. If changes to your diet and lifestyle don't improve your symptoms, it could be a sign that something more serious is going on, like endometriosis or PCOS, and that you should seek medical help.

CHAPTER 3
FINDING YOUR NORMAL

The inability to read diminishes self-esteem and opportunities to participate in the exchange of ideas. The connection to the lives of girls and women is obvious — the education of girls is a key strategy in all international development work. It struck me that most educated women in developed countries live with another kind of illiteracy — (we) are not taught to "read" or understand (our) own bodies. On the contrary, (we) are taught to distrust (our) bodies and accept various artificial means to "manage" them.

— Laura Wershler[1]

There is power in literacy, and there is power in body literacy. Learning this term, championed by Laura Wershler at the 2005 SMCR conference in Boulder, Colorado, was a pivotal moment for me. Finally, I had a way to describe the work I was piecing together that centred on menstrual health, nutrition, and holistic wellness.

Being able to read and understand the signs of your menstrual cycle is at the heart of Wershler's definition of body literacy. I want to push this idea further. Body literacy isn't something that should be limited to reproductive health; it extends well beyond our menstrual cycles — we need to be able to read and understand *all* our body's signs and signals. That doesn't mean we all need to be able to diagnose our own symptoms, but we do need to be able to *listen* to what our body is telling us — something that many of us have never been taught to do. The demands of modern society are such that we are constantly overriding our body's cues and signals. We don't rest when we're tired, we don't eat when we're hungry or stop when we're full. We're constantly looking to external sources to understand our own bodies instead of going inward and *trusting* what we hear.

We ignore our bodies at our peril.

At the same time, perhaps one of the reasons why we learn not to take our own intuition about our bodies seriously is because no one else does. I have heard countless stories of women going to doctors not feeling well or concerned about their health, only to be dismissed. An online poll by the National Pain Report found 65 percent of survey respondents felt doctors took their pain less seriously because of their sex.

Tracking your menstrual cycle requires a certain intimacy with your body. It requires that you can hear what your body is telling you, but also that you can interpret its signs and signals, something that is often easier said than done — at least in the beginning. In order to be able to accurately track your menstrual cycle, interpret it, and make any necessary changes to your nutrition and lifestyle, you first need to be in touch with your body. Before you can learn to track your cycle, you need to learn to listen to your body.

GETTING TO KNOW YOUR BODY

In order to become truly body literate, you need to do more than just look at anatomy charts. Getting to know your body means getting to know *your* body, through touch and observation. Many people, particularly those who identify as a woman, are so disconnected from their bodies that before they can even start the process of touching or looking, they need to learn how to actually *be* in their bodies. So, before you grab a mirror, start with taking a nice, deep breath.

Our modern lives have us running from one obligation to the next, with little time for quiet introspection. I'm not talking about contemplating the cosmos, just simply tuning in to our bodies and how we feel on a day-to-day basis.

You don't need to sit on a meditation cushion for an hour every day (although that is a lovely aspirational thought); you just need five minutes to take a deep breath, close your eyes, and ask yourself how you're doing. You can do this on the subway, before you turn out the light at night, in the bathroom stall at work — wherever and whenever you have five minutes. If you don't have five minutes, start with even just one! It will still make a big difference to your body literacy. It's an easy investment in your well-being that will yield big returns, yet doesn't cost a cent.

Breathe

Does this seem too simple? Maybe. But there's a good chance that you're spending a good part of the day holding your breath. What does breathing have to do with periods? The answer is, a lot, actually. And not just because your breath is linked to your stress level, which has an enormous impact on your menstrual cycle, but also because how do you expect to listen to your body and interpret the signs that it's telling you if you're not even breathing?

I suggest you sit or lie in a comfortable position and take a few deep breaths to "arrive in your body," as they say in yoga class. You don't have to worry about what's happened today or what's to come. Do a quick and easy body scan, starting from the top of your head and moving down to your toes. How does your body feel? Is anything tight or in pain? What is your energy like today? How is your digestion? Have you been to the bathroom lately? Is your stomach bloated or tied up in knots? Are you feeling tired or are you so wired it's impossible to even sit still for this exercise?

Look at this with objectivity — you're not there to judge whether what you're feeling is right or wrong. The purpose of this exercise is simply to start listening to your body. Don't worry if you're not feeling anything right away. Many of us have lived our whole lives without learning to understand the connection between our body, mind, and spirit — so it might take some practice to start to tune in. But once you do, you can use it as a powerful way to connect with your body and your menstrual cycle.

Give Yourself a Physical Examination

No need for stirrups here, just grab a mirror and take a look at yourself! What does your vulva look like? Do you know where your clitoris is in relation to your urethra and your anus? Once you've learned how to breathe and feel your body, it's a good time to actually *look* at your body. You know, with your eyes.

Women and femme-presenting people are conditioned to spend a part of their day looking in the mirror. We do our makeup, style our hair, take an outfit of the day selfie in the work bathroom's banging lighting, all while looking in the mirror. But when was the last time you really looked at your body in the mirror, if ever? Do you enjoy what you see, or is your first instinct to start pointing out your flaws? Diet culture is so rampant today that we've made it normal for women to hate their bodies. Complaining about our thighs or our bums or our arms is practically a competitive sport in many female social circles. Claiming your menstrual cycles starts with claiming your whole body and acknowledging it as the beautiful, sacred vessel that it is.

Now what about down below? While you may catch a glimpse of your naked body in the mirror every so often, you probably don't often make a concerted effort to look at your genitals. Little girls are taught that it's shameful to touch themselves "down there," and it's unlikely that you were ever encouraged to pull out a mirror and take a look at your vulva. Getting to know this part of your body is a crucial step for healing the wound of internalized misogyny. Being taught that touching yourself is gross and dirty is closely related to the menstrual taboo; menstrual products are designed so that you don't even have to touch your body to use them. Getting to know your vulva can be empowering, whether you're advocating for yourself within the medical system or you're simply looking to switch to a menstrual cup.

Take your time when it comes to getting to know your body, particularly as you explore your internal and external genitals. It's an area that can come with a lot of complicated emotions, particularly if you're a survivor of any type of sexual abuse. While checking yourself out in the mirror or through an internal cervical exam can be helpful and empowering to some, it may be triggering to others. Don't do anything that doesn't feel right to you. Go slow.

When you're ready, once you've learned how to take a deep breath and actually listen to your body, and you've taken a good, loving look at the outside of what your mama gave you, it's time to take a page from our second-wave feminist foremothers and break out the mirror, get comfy, and take a look at that beautiful cervix of yours (shag carpets are completely optional).

Internal self-exams using a speculum and mirror were popular during the women's health movement of the sixties and seventies, and for good reason — how can you understand and advocate for a part of your body that you've never even looked at before? Our relationship with our genitalia is often within the context of sex and someone else's pleasure, or a medical setting, like getting a Pap test or internal exam. I remember changing my daughter's diaper when she was just a few weeks old and realizing this was the first time I had ever seen a vulva head-on.

Beyond empowerment, there are practical reasons to take a regular look at your genitals, too. Polyps, lesions, and masses can grow in our vaginas and on our cervixes. You'd be alarmed to wake up one morning and find something growing on your elbow; the same should be true for your internal reproductive organs. Of course, self-exams aren't meant to replace your regular physical exams or Paps performed by your doctor. Think of them instead as in addition to your regular checkups.

Your cervix is closer than you think, so get to know it!

HOW TO PERFORM A CERVICAL SELF-EXAM

In her book *A New View of a Women's Body*, Carol Downer, a feminist lawyer and leader of the early women's health movement, advocated for women to give themselves a cervical self-exam. While popular during the seventies, it's not something that is often talked about today, but it's still a great way to get to know your body. All you need is a speculum and a flashlight. While Downer stole a speculum from a doctor's office in the sixties, they're now easy to buy online and often come in multipacks so you can share with a friend!

To perform the exam, get comfortable and slowly insert the speculum. Position the flashlight and mirror so you can get a good look at your cervix. Depending on where you are in your menstrual cycle, your cervix may also be positioned higher or lower in the vaginal canal, and the os, the opening in the middle, may be open to allow cervical mucus or menstrual blood to pass through, or it will be tightly closed.

Your vaginal canal and cervix will likely resemble the inside of your cheek in terms of colour and moisture. The muscles of the vagina can sometimes give the walls the appearance of being textured or rippled.

Get a good look, and then, as you get into the habit of a regular self-exam, start looking for changes in colour or shape, or any growths. If you do see a change, be sure to see your doctor right away.

GETTING TO KNOW YOUR MENSTRUAL CYCLE

When I worked in corporate communications, we had a saying: "You can't manage what you don't measure." Which was to say that if you're not monitoring what you're doing, then you have no way of knowing if you're on track or not, and perhaps more importantly, you won't be able to course-correct if needed.

The same goes for your menstrual cycle. You won't be able to tap into the insight of your cycle as a vital sign if you're not tracking it. Do you know your blood pressure at any given time? No, you need to monitor it by using a blood pressure cuff or one of those fancy machines at the pharmacy. Same goes for your menstrual cycle (although you don't need any fancy equipment for this one).

Tracking your cycle, or "charting" as it's often referred to in Fertility Awareness Methods (FAM), has a number of benefits — the most obvious being that you can predict when you're ovulating or when your next period is about to arrive.

Tracking or charting your cycle can also be used as a way to avoid or achieve pregnancy. When you are able to identify your "fertile window" — the days when you are approaching ovulation and therefore are fertile — you are able to make decisions about sex and contraception. While varying methods differ in terms of efficacy rates, symptom-thermal methods of fertility awareness that incorporate cervical mucus observation and basal body temperatures can be as effective as hormonal contraception with perfect use.[2]

And, of course, charting will also give you a window into your overall health and wellness; your menstrual cycle can reflect hormonal imbalances, nutritional deficiencies, allergies, immunological problems, and other health issues.[3] When your endocrine system is functioning well, your other body systems will too.

As Dr. Lara Briden says, when you are unwell your period will tell the story. When you are healthy and your hormones are balanced, you will be ovulating regularly and your period will show up regularly, and with minimal pain or discomfort.

When it comes to health, menstrual or otherwise, it's important to know what your normal is. As we discussed in the previous chapter, there are certainly guidelines as to what a healthy cycle looks like. But where do you fall within those guidelines? What is *your* normal? If you don't know what is normal to begin with, you won't be able to identify changes.

Say that your cycle is consistently twenty-nine days, plus or minus a day or two here and there when you may have had a busy period at work or have been travelling. You've been tracking your cycles and you notice that suddenly your cycles have jumped to around thirty-five days in length for a few cycles. You're still within the window of what is considered to be normal, but there has clearly been a change to your "normal" and that warrants further investigation.

Being able to identify a shift in your own patterns can help you advocate for yourself when talking to your doctor or other health care professionals because you'll be able to demonstrate that something has changed by showing your charts. When I see my GP for my yearly exam or whenever I begin working with a new practitioner, like a naturopath or acupuncturist, I simply export the data from my menstrual tracking apps and attach it to my intake forms to give them a big picture overview of my hormonal health.

BEYOND FERTILITY: MENSTRUAL CYCLE AWARENESS

Fertility awareness is a set of practices used to determine the fertile and infertile phases of the menstrual cycle, including checking cervical fluid and basal body temperature, then charting the data on paper or in an app. As its name implies, Fertility Awareness Methods are generally used to achieve or avoid pregnancy. While the methods differ, with perfect use and instruction by a professional, the efficacy rates of this system rival that of both hormonal contraception and condoms at 99.6 percent.[4] But these charts can tell us much more than just whether or not we're in a fertile window and ripe for pregnancy.

Reframing fertility awareness as menstrual cycle awareness takes the emphasis off fertility and baby-making and helps to attract to the practice those who don't want to have children or aren't at risk for pregnancy — such as people who don't sleep with men, or those whose male partners have had a vasectomy.

But why track your cycle if fertility isn't on your radar? Well, there are many good reasons, including the following:

- Hormonal issues such as low progesterone or issues with the thyroid can show up in a menstrual chart as short luteal phases or low body temperatures.

- Charting can help you predict when you'll get your next period.
- Overlaying a record of physical symptoms or changes in mood can help detect cyclical patterns and rule out or determine if symptoms are related to your menstrual cycle.
- Paired with a food diary, it can help to identify how foods affect your hormones and periods.
- As you get older, tracking changes to your menstrual cycle can help you determine when you're entering perimenopause.

How to Track Your Cycle

Tracking your menstrual cycle has a number of benefits, providing a window into your health, linking any recurring symptoms to your hormones, understanding when you're in your fertile phase, helping you navigate ebbs and flows in your energy levels, and, last but not least, predicting when you're likely to start your next period.

When it comes to tracking your cycle, there are a few basic things that you want to record:

- **The first day of your period.** The first day of bleeding is the first day of a new menstrual cycle. In order to know how long our cycles are, we need to know when they started! This is also helpful to know where you are in your cycle when looking for other important signs like ovulation. Any spotting leading up to your period is counted in the previous cycle. Generally, the first day you need to use a menstrual product beyond a liner is the first day of your period.
- **Your period.** How long is your period and how much are you bleeding? Record if your period is heavy, light, or somewhere in between. You may also want to note any noticeable changes that you observe, like the sudden appearance of large clots or a change in consistency or colour.
- **Cervical fluid/mucus.** As you move through the follicular phase of your cycle, estrogen levels begin to rise and form cervical mucus as you approach ovulation. This fluid is produced by your cervix and helps to move sperm through the uterus and up into the ovarian tubes for fertilization. It changes in colour, texture, and volume during your cycle. Tracking can

help you determine when you're in your fertile window and if you are ovulating.

- **Cervical positioning.** Your cervix also goes through several changes during your menstrual cycle that can be helpful in determining your fertile window and getting to know your cycle. This is considered to be an optional sign in many Fertility Awareness Methods, but tracking cervical position can be a good practice when you're just getting to know your body and learning to interpret your cycle. When you are bleeding, it is soft and open to allow menstrual blood to flow through the vagina; and when you are in your ovulation phase, this is how sperm enters into the uterus to reach the ovarian tubes. Outside of your period and fertile window, your cervix is higher up in the vaginal canal, closed, and feels hard, kind of like the tip of your nose. Get to know your cervix! Tracking its position will also help to identify where you are in your menstrual cycle and if you might be ovulating.

- **Basal body temperature.** Your body temperature shifts slightly in your luteal phase following ovulation, thanks to progesterone, which makes the body warmer. While the only way to truly confirm ovulation is through ultrasound, tracking your temperature can be a good clue that you've ovulated. Following ovulation, your chart should show a slight, upward shift in your temperature, and it will stay high until progesterone falls, which is when you can expect your period. If you're pregnant, your temperature will remain high throughout pregnancy. If your temperature has stayed high for longer than two weeks, you may be pregnant. Consistently low temperatures may be an indication of thyroid imbalances. The trick is you need to take your temperature first thing in the morning– that means before you get out of bed, take a sip of water or even start talking — after at least four hours of uninterrupted sleep.

Other Things to Track

Once you understand how to observe and chart the basic signs of fertility, you can layer on other symptoms like PMS and pain to discover how they sync up with your cycle. You might be surprised that recurring symptoms are occurring at the same time in your cycle every month. It's possible to have recurring symptoms that are related to hormones at any point during your cycle, not just during the PMS window.

If you are tracking PMS symptoms such as breast tenderness, changes in mood, headaches, pain, or others, record when they start and the length and severity of the pain or condition.

You can also record travel, exercise, intercourse — anything that you think would be valuable for understanding your hormonal and overall health picture.

Tools and Resources for Menstrual Cycle Awareness

It doesn't take much to track your menstrual cycles and fertility signs. There are all kinds of apps out there today, or, if you prefer, you can go analogue with paper and a pencil.

Mark the days of your cycle and any symptoms on a calendar, in a journal, or on a chart specifically for fertility charting — there are many blank charts available for download on the internet (refer to the resources at the end of this book for where to find them).

Tracking your menstrual cycles? There's an app for that! There are countless period tracking apps out there, but they are certainly *not* created equal. The majority of apps available are designed only for tracking your periods, which is not the same as tracking your menstrual cycle. Many of these algorithms are based solely on the first day of your last period and don't account for your fertile signs. Tracking your ovulation is just as important as tracking your period, if not more so! And not just if you're trying to get pregnant. After all, ovulation is what we get all those amazing health benefits from.

If you want to use an app to track your cycle, make sure that you find one created specifically for fertility awareness charting. These apps aren't just for logging your period, but also for recording the other signs of fertility outlined in the previous section, such as basal body temperature, cervical mucus, and positioning. Some fertility awareness apps have even introduced digital Bluetooth thermometers that automatically sync your basal body temperature with the other signs and information that you're tracking.

Without these signs, an app isn't truly able to make an accurate prediction of ovulation and therefore is unreliable for avoiding or achieving pregnancy. Many of these apps are not designed for body literacy.

IS YOUR PERIOD LATE?

Here's the thing about your period: it can never be late. It will always show up right on time, which is about two weeks after you've ovulated. Recall that the luteal phase of your menstrual cycle is finite; it can only last up to 14–16 days. Although low progesterone or hormonal imbalance can certainly make the luteal phase shorter than this, it's impossible for it to be any longer given that the corpus luteum can only survive for about two weeks. However, your follicular phase can vary from cycle to cycle. It's normal for it to vary by a day or two each month, but it can be delayed even longer if you're experiencing a lot of stress. So, if your period isn't showing up when you expect it, look back to when you normally would have ovulated to see what might have been going on that would delay ovulation — stress, illness, poor nutrition, and travel can all inhibit ovulation.

Like many apps that have become part of our daily lives, they are free to use. But that doesn't mean that we're not paying for them in some way; more often than not it's with our data. The data that we input into period or fertility tracking apps may be sold to third-party companies or used to target advertising. Something to consider when looking for an app to track your menstrual cycles — or any app really — is what kind of data you will be inputting and how the company behind it is going to use that data. Make sure to review the app maker's privacy policies before signing up.

I would also be remiss if I let you think that you can outsource your body literacy entirely to an app — this shouldn't be a set-it-and-forget-it scenario, especially if you're depending on using this information to avoid a pregnancy. Apps are only a tool that you can use to understand your body and inform your decision making; they should not replace ongoing observation of your menstrual cycle, nor should they replace training from a qualified professional who can help read and interpret your body signs.

There are various methods of fertility awareness, and each one varies a little bit in terms of what and how they track, and what the "rules" are when it comes to fertile windows. What I've outlined here are just the basics — and while it should be more than enough to get you started with menstrual cycle awareness, there are many nuances involved when using a Fertility Awareness Method to achieve pregnancy or for birth control. Regardless of your objectives for using FAM, I recommend checking out the resources section at the end of this book for recommendations on where to learn more and seeking out a qualified reproductive health practitioner for one-on-one guidance as you learn to chart and interpret your cycles.

INTERPRETING YOUR CYCLE

Once you've begun collecting data around your menstrual cycle and health, it's time to learn how to interpret it. What should you be looking for, and how do you find it?

Give yourself at least three months of charting before you dive in to analyzing the data. This should give you enough time to establish a baseline of your normal and to notice any patterns or draw any links between symptoms and your hormones.

Here are a few things to look out for in your charts when you start interpreting your cycles:

- The length of your complete cycle
- The length of your period and how heavy your flow is each day
- If you have any spotting leading up to your period in the last half of your luteal phase
- When your fertile window opens and closes based on cervical mucus variations and body temperature shifts
- Any symptoms that might occur around the same point of your cycle month after month (even if symptoms are falling outside of your PMS window, they may still be linked to hormonal fluctuations)
- How certain foods impact your cycles
- The effect of travel, illness, or stress factors

Consider learning how to chart and interpret your cycles from an experienced fertility awareness educator or holistic reproductive health practitioner who can teach you to read and understand the signals your body is expressing through your menstrual cycle.

CHAPTER 4
WHEN GOOD PERIODS GO BAD

Suffering due to pain or psychological symptoms associated with your period is pretty common, if not the norm — anywhere from about half to almost 95 percent of menstruators report some type of physical or psychological discomfort before or during their periods.

However, just because period pain and other unpleasant menstrual symptoms are common, that does not make them normal.

For some reason — *ahem*, gender bias, *ahem* — menstrual pain is the only pain that's considered to be par for the course! When someone experiences pain in any other part of their body, it's considered to be a sign that something is wrong; in fact, some medical professionals once considered pain itself to be a vital sign. This is no longer the case because pain is subjective and therefore difficult to measure consistently, but that old practice still demonstrates the importance that pain plays in the body.

Despite being such a common occurrence, PMS and other conditions that cause pain and discomfort before or during the menstrual cycle aren't hot topics for medical research. The fact that pain is so common might even be the reason why it's not studied — in other words, it's never occurred to researchers to look into it because it's so pervasive.[1] An early educational pamphlet published by a menstrual product company even stated that it was the woman who *didn't* experience any negative side effects of menstruation that was the exception, not the norm.

Depending on the symptoms and your overall health picture, the underlying causes of period-related symptoms can vary, from hormonal imbalances to nutrient deficiencies, or other underlying health concerns such as an under- or overactive thyroid. According to one study, many chronic illnesses, such as diabetes, epilepsy, or migraine headaches, are exacerbated during the premenstrual window[2] — the week leading up to your period.

And while pain may be common, that doesn't mean nothing can be done about it. Many women have suffered, perhaps needlessly, for years because of a lack of treatment options available to them, or because the shame of the menstrual taboo keeps them from discussing these issues with their doctors. Given that hormones are so sensitive to nutrition and lifestyle, there's actually a lot that can be done to improve your period experience and make it less of a "curse."

Here's a look at some of the common period problems and what's behind them. We'll then take a look at how food and lifestyle factors, like stress, affect your period.

Premenstrual Syndrome (PMS)

PMS refers to a number of both physical and psychological symptoms associated with the luteal phase — the time between ovulation and the onset of menstruation. The diagnostic manual classifies around 150 various symptoms related to PMS, including abdominal bloating, acne, anxiety, backache, breast swelling and tenderness, cramps, depression, food cravings, fainting, fatigue, headaches, insomnia, joint pain, nervousness, pimples and other skin eruptions, water retention, and personality changes ranging from drastic mood swings to outbursts of anger, violence, and thoughts of suicide (in very severe cases).

Interestingly, PMS, formerly known as premenstrual tension, first entered the diagnostic manual in 1954, just two years after "hysteria," once a common psychiatric diagnosis for women, was removed. A few of the symptoms of hysteria included irritability, bloating, heaviness in the abdomen, and insomnia — all of which are now classified under PMS.

But while PMS was formally recognized as a disorder in the 1950s, it really wasn't until the early eighties that it gained public recognition. In fact, it was poised to be the "disease of the 1980s" until HIV — a real disease — became a crisis.

While there are no hard statistics, it's estimated that 80 percent of those of us who get our period experience PMS. About 5 percent describe their symptoms as incapacitating and another 30 to 40 percent say their PMS interferes with their daily lives.[3] As a result of the stigma associated with menstruation and the lack of research around its causes, the extent to which premenstrual disorders impact our lives is under-recognized by pretty much everyone, including medical doctors, governments, health organizations, and even the people who are experiencing it.

The cause of PMS isn't clear — perhaps because it may have a different root cause for different people — and there isn't even a general consensus on how to diagnose it. Because of this, and because the symptoms that fall under the PMS umbrella are so broad, there isn't a clear and reliable method of treatment, either.[4] It's possible that there are multiple causes of PMS and that different causes affect different people.

There is also no standardized way to test for PMS. If you were to compare the hormone levels of those of us who experience PMS and those who don't, they would be virtually indistinguishable.[5] Because of this, medical practitioners rely on patients providing retrospective data — essentially recalling symptoms from previous cycles — in order to assess symptoms. The problem with that, though, is that as humans we're just not that great when it comes to remembering what our previous experiences were like, particularly when it comes to our periods. This is highlighted in the dramatic placebo response in studies related to PMS. *Any* treatment seems to have a positive effect because it seems that we always recall our last periods as being the worst.

As a nutritionist, I am particularly interested in the role that diet may play in PMS, which has been linked to food allergies, changes in carbohydrate metabolism, hypoglycemia (blood sugar regulation), and nutrient malabsorption. A number of vitamin and mineral deficiencies, especially of calcium, have been shown to contribute to premenstrual symptoms.[6]

Heavy Flow

The official name for a heavy menstrual flow is menorrhagia. Officially, more than eighty millilitres of menstrual blood flowing over the course of the entire period — that's about sixteen soaked pads or tampons — classifies as a heavy flow.

But according to the Centre for Menstrual Cycle and Ovulation Research (CeMCOR) in Vancouver, menstrual flows can range from a spot to over two cups. Individuals who are taller, have had children, or are experiencing perimenopause have the heaviest flows. Endometriosis, a serious disease that affects the reproductive system, is also marked by heavy menstrual bleeding.

How much you're actually bleeding on your period can be difficult to discern, particularly if you're using tampons or pads that absorb your flow. You might think that you have a heavy flow when really you're within what's considered to be normal, and many people who report heavy periods are actually within this normal, if not light, range. It goes the other way, too — 40 percent of those who had menstrual blood loss that qualified as excessive uterine bleeding reporting having normal, even light, periods![7]

Soaking through pads or tampons or having an overflowing menstrual cup that needs to be changed several times a day definitely constitutes a heavy flow. If this is the case, you don't need to have an exact volume measurement in order to qualify for a heavy flow diagnosis.

But if you're simply curious or interested in knowing where you land, pay attention next time you're on your period. It can be difficult to measure your flow when using tampons or pads. Because of the risk of toxic shock syndrome and infection, you might need to change a pad or tampon before it has been fully soaked through. For this reason, I recommend using a menstrual cup, particularly one that includes volume markers, to determine exactly how much fluid you're losing during your flow.

While it's not yet perfectly clear what the cause of heavy menstrual bleeding is, it's most common in adolescence and perimenopause when estrogen is higher and progesterone is lower. Therefore, it's possible that estrogen levels that are too high can contribute to heavy bleeding or "flooding" periods. Many people who experience heavy periods also have uterine fibroids — benign tumors — but it seems that this is rarely the cause of the bleeding and simply a coincidence.

Painful Periods

Menstrual cramps are the most common gynecological problem in young adolescent menstruators, with some studies reporting that anywhere from 16 to 91 percent of them experience cramps that cause missed school days or the need for pain medication each month.[8] While cramps, known medically as dysmenorrhea, do appear to taper off after adolescence (once the menstrual cycle has reached maturation) or after pregnancy,[9] there are still plenty of people in their premenopause years who experience cramps and pain associated with their periods.

This pain is caused by prostaglandins, a hormone-like substance found in the walls of the uterus. These prostaglandins cause the uterus to contract, which not only contributes to menstrual cramps but also contractions during pregnancy release. High levels of estrogen and a tight lining of the uterus contribute to higher levels of prostaglandins. The more prostaglandins we have, the more cramping we may experience.

And since prostaglandins are also a part of the body's inflammatory response, inflammation may also contribute to increased period pain. As such, reducing our inflammation can help alleviate period pain. We'll cover how to do that in the coming chapters on nutrition.

Breast Pain

Mastalgia, the medical term for breast pain, can be cyclical and related to hormones — showing up as breast tenderness or pain before and during your period. Like cramping, we have prostaglandins to thank for this one, too. Progesterone released following ovulation stimulates ducts in the breasts to begin milk production and prostaglandins trigger an inflammatory response for ducts to swell up to make room for milk in the event of a pregnancy.

Higher levels of estrogen that are unopposed by progesterone can contribute to breast tenderness. If you have tender breasts before or during your period, promoting ovulation, and therefore the production of progesterone, can help to relieve symptoms.

Headaches and Migraines

More than half of people with periods report menstrual-related headaches and migraines.[10] Sensitivity to hormonal fluctuations can trigger a headache or migraine and it can occur at any point of your cycle, not just in the PMS window. Keeping a diary of your headaches and migraines alongside tracking your menstrual cycles can help to draw a link between the pain and hormones. Certain foods may also trigger headaches and migraines, so you may also want to keep a food diary alongside tracking your cycles and headaches.

Long Cycles

What if you're getting your period regularly, but you fall outside of the thirty-five days window? The medical term for long cycles is oligomenorrhea, and it is classified as a cycle that is longer than thirty-five days, but still shorter than 180 (anything over 180 days is classified as amenorrhea, or an absence of menstruation). Generally, long cycles can be attributed to an underlying condition such as polycystic ovarian syndrome (PCOS), which will delay or impair ovulation, lengthening your cycles.

Irregular Cycles

In my experience, many people report "irregular cycles" to be outside of the "regular" twenty-eight days — misunderstanding that the window of what's "normal" actually falls a week on either side of twenty-eight days. Another common misconception about the menstrual cycle is that it has to be the same length every month. Not true — given hormonal sensitivity to lifestyle factors like stress and illness, it's normal for there to be some fluctuation from cycle to cycle, plus or minus a few days.

Truly irregular cycles have a wide variation from cycle to cycle — for instance a thirty-five-day cycle followed by a ninety-day cycle. There is generally an underlying condition like PCOS that is inhibiting ovulation and contributing to the irregularity.

Mittelschmerz

German for "mid pain," *mittelschmerz* is the medical term for painful ovulation. For some, it may be dull and cramp-like, while others experience mittelschmerz as a sharp, sudden, "stabbing" pain. It usually occurs on one side at a time, depending on which ovary is releasing the egg, and may be accompanied by spotting or light bleeding. You might experience mittelschmerz every month or every once in a while. Interestingly, I experience mittelschmerz, but only ever on my left side!

Amenorrhea

There are two types of amenorrhea, which is the absence of a period — primary, meaning that menstruation hasn't started by age sixteen, and secondary, which is when you have had a period but not for about five months. Illness, intense exercise, eating disorders, and chronic stress are all contributing factors to amenorrhea. Amenorrhea experienced after stopping hormonal contraception is known as post-pill amenorrhea. Breastfeeding can also suppress ovulation and cause a period of amenorrhea postpartum.

Fibroids

Fibroids are benign growths in the uterus, made from tissue that is white, hard, and gristly, like high-density plastic.[11] They are common in most females over the age of thirty-five — anywhere from 20 percent to 50 percent of females have fibroids, and black women are three to nine times more likely than white women to develop them.

While fibroids generally do not cause any symptoms and are discovered only during a routine pelvic exam, many people suffer a great deal because of fibroids. The presence of fibroids may contribute to pelvic discomfort, frequent urination, or back pain. Occasionally the uterus tries to expel a fibroid, which causes intense pain similar to that of labour. It's not unusual to also experience heavy menstrual bleeding along with fibroids, but research suggests that this has more to do with both conditions being linked to estrogen excess than fibroids causing bleeding. Despite being the number one reason for hysterectomies in people aged forty-five to fifty-four,[12] fibroids don't generally need surgery or treatment and usually resolve by menopause. Natural treatments such as changes to diet or lifestyle won't make fibroids go away but can help to make them stop growing or prevent new ones forming.

Cysts

A benign growth on the ovary is known as a cyst. There are several different types of cysts. They can be completely asymptomatic and go away on their own, or they may cause a feeling of fullness or pressure in the abdomen, pain, nausea, or bleeding. Cysts can rupture, which can cause bleeding and pain that lasts anywhere from a few hours to a few days. Occasionally cysts may be very large and require surgery. Oviducts can get twisted under the weight of a large cyst, which is very painful and requires medical attention, as does the rupture of a cyst. Most small cysts will go away on their own. Although hormonal contraception is commonly prescribed as a treatment for cysts, it won't make any existing cysts go away and will only prevent the formation of new cysts.

Adenomyosis

Sometimes referred to as "internal endometriosis," adenomyosis is a contributing factor in very painful or heavy periods. The endometrium breaks through the muscle walls of the uterus, growing inward instead of out into the uterine cavity, causing "knots" of lining to form in the muscles. It is very painful during menstruation as the spongy walls of the uterus fill with blood. In addition to the pain and heavy bleeding, a distended abdomen is another common symptom. Adenomyosis can only be diagnosed using MRI or biopsy and is generally treated with hysterectomy.

WHEN IT'S NOT JUST A "BAD PERIOD" BUT SOMETHING MORE SERIOUS

There are times when symptoms related to menstruation or the menstrual cycle are more than just a bad period. There are a number of diseases that are not necessarily hormonal diseases but are linked to period pain or other menstrual-related symptoms. Diseases like endometriosis or premenstrual dysphoric disorder may be expressed around your period but are serious diseases that should be treated as such. Bleeding disorders like hemophilia or Von Willebrand disease can also be expressed as very heavy bleeding and long periods. Another thing to be aware of is that hormonal fluctuations may worsen the symptoms of other diseases that have nothing to do with your menstrual cycle. Keeping track of your cycles and your symptoms can help to identify any links.

Below is some information about a few of the more common diseases that affect menstruation.

Premenstrual Dysphoric Disorder

When the psychological symptoms of PMS like depression and anxiety are extreme, combined with violence and suicidal ideation, it is classified as premenstrual dysphoric disorder (PMDD), which is a mental illness and requires the appropriate care and medication that comes with such a diagnosis.

Polycystic Ovarian Syndrome (PCOS)

It's estimated that as many as one in ten suffer from polycystic ovarian syndrome (PCOS). PCOS is not one disease,[13] and symptoms vary from person to person, but can include irregular periods, amenorrhea, elevated levels of male hormones (androgens), acne, excess facial hair, and infertility. Polycystic ovaries have multiple small cysts covering them. These cysts differ from larger ovarian cysts and do not cause pain. It's not uncommon to have "polycystic ovaries" at certain points during their cycle. Because of this, PCOS can't be diagnosed just from ultrasound. It's not enough to just have polycystic ovaries, although plenty have been diagnosed this way (including myself), which may contribute to misdiagnosis of PCOS. The Androgen Excess Society's diagnostic criteria states that a patient must also have elevated levels of androgens in order to qualify for a PCOS diagnosis.

Other guidelines only need two of the following criteria in order to make a diagnosis of PCOS:

- Irregular periods
- Elevated levels of androgens
- Polycystic ovaries

Given the variety of symptoms, there are also a variety of contributing factors to PCOS, including hormonal birth control, hormonal imbalance, insulin resistance, and inflammation.

Endometriosis

Endometriosis is an inflammatory disease that causes cells similar to the lining of the uterus, the endometrium, to grow outside of the uterus on other parts of the body, such as the ovaries, bowel, and other organs. It's difficult to diagnose without surgery. At least one in ten suffer from endometriosis, and while it is not specifically a disease of the reproductive system, it often affects a woman's menstrual cycle, contributing to "bad periods." Symptoms can include extremely heavy periods, severe cramping, pain, digestive problems, urinary incontinence, depression, and anxiety — and symptoms aren't necessarily confined to your PMS window or your period. Endometriosis is frequently treated with hormones or hysterectomy — although neither guarantees that symptoms won't return. There is emerging evidence that endometriosis isn't a hormonal disease but rather an inflammatory condition or autoimmune disease. While there is no cure for endometriosis, many patients find that diet and lifestyle changes and alternative modalities can help to manage symptoms.

CHAPTER 5

YOUR PERIOD QUESTIONS ANSWERED

Despite having had your period for years, maybe even decades, it's understandable that you might still have questions about what's happening with your cycle given that so many of us lack an in-depth education about our menstrual cycles beyond which products to use. Now that you have a better understanding of how the menstrual cycle works, what's normal and what's not, you still might have some questions about some of the more, shall we say, *finer* points of having a menstrual cycle.

Here I've tried to answer some of the most frequently asked questions I've received about menstrual cycles, from sex to skin and everything in between.

Why Does My Period Mess with My Skin?

Estrogen, progesterone, and testosterone all have an influence on the health and appearance of your skin. Estrogen helps to keep your skin smooth and hydrated, while progesterone tightens up your pores and contributes to your skin's "glow" — it's the high levels of progesterone during pregnancy that give pregnant people great skin. Testosterone increases sebum production, which can lead to acne and breakouts.

At the start of your cycle, when you're on your period, estrogen and progesterone are both low. During this time, you might have lingering breakouts or blemishes that cropped up during your PMS week and your skin might be a little dull as a result of these low hormone levels.

The middle of your cycle is likely when your skin will look its best, when estrogen and progesterone are both at their peak. Then, before your next period, these hormones fall while testosterone remains high. Progesterone tightens up your pores and the sebum that's produced by testosterone can get trapped under the skin, leading to breakouts.

These hormone-related breakouts tend to crop up on your jaw line and cheeks. If you're breaking out in the same places around the same point of your cycle month after month, it's a good sign that there's a hormonal component to your acne.

Do Menstrual Cycles Sync Up?

It seems like just about everyone has a story about their cycles syncing up with their work wife, a roommate, partner, or friend. But is it true?

In 1971, Harvard psychologist Martha McClintock published a paper titled "Menstrual Synchronicity and Suppression," which looked at the menstrual cycles of 135 young women living in a college dormitory. The study found the evidence for synchronicity to be quite strong and suggested that there is a physiological process that affects menstrual cycles. McClintock theorized that pheromones, a chemical substance the human body produces and releases into the environment, caused the menstrual cycles to sync up.

However, since the original study was published, it has been criticized for its research methods. Subsequent studies have been unable to replicate the findings — for every study that finds cycles do sync up, there's another one that doesn't.

In 2017, Clue, the period tracking app, partnered with Oxford University to find out if menstrual cycles actually sync up. The study looked at 360 pairs of women and found that cycles between pairs and cohabiting individuals did not align. In fact, the results even indicated the opposite — that over time, cycles are actually more likely to diverge.

If cycles do overlap, it's likely more to do with chance. The average length of a menstrual cycle and period varies widely: by as much as two weeks.

Despite the fact that there appears to be no scientific basis for cycle syncing, the idea persists. We really *want* to believe that our cycles sync up — a study published in 1999 revealed that 80 percent of survey respondents believed that menstrual cycles sync up and 70 percent enjoyed the phenomenon. I know that I always get a little warm and fuzzy feeling when my cycle syncs up with a friend — or, say, every female cousin and aunt that I travelled to Las Vegas with for a family trip back in 2004.

While we're no longer isolated in menstrual huts, the experience of menstruation can still be pretty isolating because we're supposed to keep the details to ourselves. A study from 2014 concluded that the belief in menstrual synchronicity enhances gender solidarity by reducing shame and taboo related to menstruation, constructing a socially acceptable modern "sisterhood," marks a woman's relationship to nature, and also aids in fighting back against sexist assumptions about menstruation and menstruating women.[1]

Does the Moon Affect My Period?

In the same vein, many also believe that our cycles are synced with or influenced by the moon and lunar cycle. However, despite the average length of a menstrual cycle and the lunar month being the same length — twenty-nine and a half days — the moon doesn't influence our periods or cycles.

An oft-cited menstrual myth is that at one time all females menstruated in sync with the moon, with their periods arriving around the time of the full moon and ovulation at the new moon. Those who believe this myth blame the artificial light of modern cities for interrupting the connection between our menstrual cycles and the moon. While there is evidence that artificial light affects our hormones,[2] if our menstrual cycles were connected with the moon, then 29.5 wouldn't just be the average — it would be the same for every person on Earth with a menstrual cycle, never wavering. But as we've seen, it's normal for a cycle to vary by a day or two from cycle to cycle. This idea also doesn't account for postpartum amenorrhea, miscarriages, or the perimenopause transition.

Sally King, director of the website Menstrual Matters, lived for several months in a remote village in South Africa without electricity, yet her "twenty-one- to twenty-four-day cycle remained unaltered and people menstruated at various times of the month, just as they do everywhere else in the world!"

A study that looked at the women of the Dogon village in Mali — a village with no electrical lighting, where women spend most nights outdoors — concluded that there was no lunar influence on menstrual cycles.[3]

Imagery associated with the moon has long been a symbol of female goddesses, reinforcing the idea that the moon holds influence over the menstrual cycle. The sun is often associated with male gods — it's hot and strong, in control of the seasons. The moon, on the other hand, is cold and wet and shines at night when we're asleep and therefore fearful of attack or supernatural forces like ghosts and vampires. These symbols only naturalize sexist beliefs about the differences between the sexes.

The same way that we want to believe that our cycles sync with a friend or colleague, the idea that there is a lunar connection to our menstrual cycles is also compelling. It's a way to connect with nature, and perhaps a bigger, unexplainable source of energy.

Even when we know how the menstrual cycle works and why, it still seems to retain an element of mysticism — something that a connection to the moon would explain.

Should I Avoid Sex While On My Period?

Period sex comes with its own special brand of taboo, as it's steeped in the respective shame of both menstruation and sexuality. Combine the sex taboo with the idea that menstrual blood is unclean or impure, and you get a potent dose of shame. Even some of the earliest writings about menstrual taboos address the topic of period sex.

My personal favourite menstrual myth dates all the way back to Pliny the Elder, who, in 77 CE, cautioned hunters from fornicating with a menstruating woman, particularly under a full moon, as the prey would sense that they had done so and stay away, making the hunt unsuccessful.

While I'm certainly no expert when it comes to hunting, I'm pretty sure that this is completely untrue. While Pliny espoused his views on period sex almost two thousand years ago, the idea that period sex is dangerous, unclean, gross, or even just plain wrong or immoral prevails today. A 2016 online survey conducted by Flex, makers of menstrual discs, found that 45 percent of people were grossed out by period sex.

Certainly, we are all entitled to our sexual preferences, but if you're grossed out by period sex, ask yourself why. It's not as if bodily fluids aren't a part of sexual activity, so what's different about menstrual blood?

And of course, that taboo around period sex focuses on the singular, hetero-normative idea that sex is a penis in a vagina. There are all kinds of ways to have sex that don't involve that particular activity.

There are no health or safety reasons why you can't have sex during menstruation. So, when it comes to period sex, the decision of whether or not to engage is really only up to your personal preference and that of your partner. There's no reason why you shouldn't, and in fact there are lots of reasons why you *should*, not the least of which is that menstrual blood makes for a great lubricant. Many find that their arousal is also heightened around the time of their period, particularly around day three, when their estrogen starts rising. The increased blood flow and activity in the nerve endings in your pelvis during menstruation can also heighten your sensitivity, which can make you feel more aroused. If pain is an issue with menstruation, orgasm releases endorphins, which act as a natural pain reliever and may help to lessen any cramping or pain that you're experiencing.

If your partner isn't down with period sex, the inward focus of menstruation is also a great time to explore your own sexuality and self-pleasure. If you're concerned about the mess, throw down a towel or hit the shower. Menstrual discs have been designed specifically with mess-free period pleasure in mind. Unlike a menstrual cup, which is cone-shaped and is held in place by the muscles within the vaginal canal, a menstrual disc is flat and sits in the fornix, behind the pubic bone where the vagina and cervix meet. This is the widest part of the vagina. While the menstrual disc will collect blood and fluid, it's not a form of contraception.

Using a menstrual cup can also help to contain the mess, although you might want to stick to exterior, non-penetrative stimulation when using a cup, given that it doesn't leave a lot of room in the vaginal canal. Although there are plenty of people out there who claim to have great sex while using a menstrual cup, this is definitely an at-your-own risk kind of situation.

The other thing to keep in mind when you're having sex while you're on your period is that you still need to take the necessary precautions to protect yourself from STIs and pregnancy — menstrual blood masks cervical fluid, making it difficult to know if you're in your fertile window.

Can You Get Pregnant On Your Period?

Whether or not you can get pregnant on your period may seem like a simple question, but it has a more complex answer that depends on cycle length, how many days you bleed, when you ovulate, and the timing of intercourse.

Menstrual blood masks the appearance of cervical mucus, making it impossible to use it as an indicator of fertility. Ovulation doesn't necessarily occur on the same day cycle to cycle, so knowing your fertile window is crucial. If you have a short overall menstrual cycle and a long period, it's entirely possible that menstruation will overlap with the progression of cervical mucus and your fertile window. Under the right conditions, that is, fertile cervical mucus, sperm can live inside the vagina and uterus for as long as five days.

In other words, you need to know your own cycle.

Despite this, the general messaging in sex education is that pregnancy can occur at any day of your cycle. While I understand the zero-risk approach is necessary for some people — teenagers, for example — the condescending tone of this messaging is that menstrual cycles are too difficult to understand or figure out, so don't even bother. When we tell young people that they can do anything, are we actually telling them that they can do anything … except for understanding their own bodies?

Learning to chart and understand your menstrual cycle under the guidance of an experienced, certified fertility awareness educator can help you determine where your fertile window lies and whether or not it's likely that you'll get pregnant while menstruating.

What's the Deal with Period Poops?

If you've ever experienced any kind of digestive upset before or during your period, you *know* what I'm talking about. This is because the prostaglandins that are acting on your uterus to contract in order to shed the lining aren't exactly, shall we say, picky about where they go. Since our intestines are so close to the uterus, our bowels are also going to be affected by the prostaglandins that are acting on the uterus. The result is period poops — diarrhea or loose stools during our menses. Reducing our inflammation in order to reduce our prostaglandins can help, as can laying off the chia pudding.

♦ PART 2 ♦
THE CURE FOR "THE CURSE"

CHAPTER 6
GETTING THE CARE
YOU DESERVE

The common idea that period pain is normal, and that nothing can be done about it, is perhaps the menstrual myth with the most damaging, far-reaching effects. Many people suffer in silence because they believe that pain is just par for the course.

Period pain and other symptoms related to the menstrual cycle are real and deserve to be treated as such. As we have discovered in earlier chapters of this book, having your pain or period experience taken seriously by medical professionals can be challenging. So, this section of the book, which is dedicated to the practical applications of improving your period, starts with a guide to advocating for yourself at the doctor's office. Here you will find practical tips for talking to your doctor, understanding your lab results, and learning how to navigate a system that is designed to deny your experience. Then we will discuss the practical applications of diet and lifestyle changes for supporting your hormonal health and improving your period experience. The effects of nutrition and exercise on PMS and other period-related symptoms have been well documented, and many people find their symptoms decrease after changing what they eat or starting a new exercise routine.

As a nutritionist, I firmly believe that food has the power to contribute to or take away from our health, but I am also realistic about its effects — both positive and negative. There are situations where no amounts of green juice or kale salads are going to cure your disease. If, after making changes to food and lifestyle, you are still experiencing period pain or other symptoms related to your menstrual cycle, it's a sign that something more serious may be at play.

In this section we will also look at the broad range of alternative and paramedical practitioners that have filled the menstrual gap in the conventional medical system and are well-suited for addressing hormonal health and period-related concerns.

SELF-ADVOCACY AT THE DOCTOR'S OFFICE

Because of gender bias, it can be challenging at best — an absolute nightmare, at worst — to navigate the medical system when you are experiencing painful periods or other symptoms related to the menstrual cycle. Chances are, if you are suffering because of your menstrual cycle — whether that's from a serious disorder like endometriosis, infertility, or just irregular periods or PMS — you are going to have to learn to be your own best advocate.

The conventional biomedical system does not look at the body from a holistic perspective. This is evident in the prevalent attitude that the menstrual cycle is only valuable in the context of fertility, as if there was not a single other reason why this bodily function would exist or have a positive effect on health outside of reproduction. Rather than look at the body holistically — including the mind and the spirit — conventional medicine is based on a system of problems and solutions. Doctors are trained to look for holes and when they find one, they plug it with medicine. If they can't find a hole that can be fixed, you are generally SOL.

Ironically, while I was writing this book, my own cycles suddenly doubled in length. I went to my doctor to investigate, and when all of my blood work came back within lab range — a common occurrence for those experiencing hormonal imbalances — there wasn't much else that she could do for me.

Our conversation went something like this:

"Your blood work came back and everything is looking normal."

"Okay, but that still doesn't explain why my cycles have doubled in length!"

"Are you thinking of getting pregnant again?"

"Not at the moment, no."

"Well, there's not much we can do then."

Because I wasn't planning on having a baby any time soon, the issues with my menstrual cycle simply weren't of interest to the doctor — there was no other context for the "hole" than fertility, and if I wasn't interested in trying to get pregnant it meant that there was no drug to plug the hole.

I'm a classic Libra, so I can see these situations from both sides. I believe that, most of the time, doctors are doing the best that they can with the knowledge that they have. The concept of the menstrual cycle as a vital sign isn't yet well known, and conventional medicine doesn't teach health from a holistic perspective.

From a patient perspective, though, this can be an incredibly frustrating experience. You don't feel well, and yet your lab results suggest otherwise. Perhaps this is when you start to wonder if it's all in your head? And so, the cycle of discounting pain and making women prove that they are sick continues.

If you are suffering because of your period, or for any reason really, let me tell you this: your pain is real. Your experience is valid. Just because symptoms are caused by your hormones doesn't mean that they are all in your head. Learning how to care for yourself and be your own best advocate within the medical system can help you be seen and heard, and hopefully lead to relief from your suffering.

Here are a few tips that can help you advocate for yourself within a medical setting to help you navigate the system and demand the attention that you deserve.

How to Talk to Your Doctor

Even if you're planning on seeing a functional medicine or paramedical practitioner, a conversation with your doctor should still be your first step. A medical doctor can help to make a clear diagnosis and rule out anything serious like endometriosis or PMDD. Other practitioners may not be able to request blood labs or imaging such as ultrasounds, which are crucial for getting a clear picture of your overall health. Depending on where you live, you may have to pay out of pocket for these expenses when working with a health care provider who isn't an MD.

Talking to your doctor about your period or menstrual cycle isn't always easy — the menstrual taboo is strong, and it can feel strange or weird to talk about your period with anyone, even if that person is a doctor. Many doctors don't yet recognize your menstrual cycle as a vital sign and automatically reach for a prescription pad to write you a script for hormonal birth control at the first mention of painful, irregular, or heavy periods — a solution that doesn't work for everyone and isn't without its own risks and consequences. But period pain is real pain and it deserves to be treated as such. If birth control isn't something that you're interested in, you still deserve to have your concerns taken seriously, and there may be other options available to you as we will discuss in the following chapters. Here are a few tips for talking to your doctor about your periods:

- **Write down specifics.** Try to be as accurate as you can about the symptoms that you're experiencing and write them down as they're happening — that way you won't forget any particular details. You don't need to have a medical degree to relay your symptoms, but accuracy is important. There is a big difference between pain in your vagina and pain on your vulva.

- **Have some data.** The first thing that a doctor, or even an alternative practitioner like a naturopath or nutritionist, is going to want to see is a record of your symptoms over at least two to three cycles. Start tracking your symptoms as soon as you can so that you can show the cyclical nature of your symptoms and identify how they link up with your menstrual cycle. Many apps allow you to export data so you can print a copy to show your doctor.

- **Phrase your concerns as questions.** Your doctor may be more receptive if you phrase your concerns as questions. Rather than coming in and saying that you read a blog post about a thyroid disease and you think you might have it, a better way to voice your concerns is to phrase it as a question. Instead ask, "Has my thyroid been tested?"

- **Have your alternative practitioner write a letter.** If you're working with an alternative practitioner and they want to request blood tests or labs that they aren't able to order for you, have them write a letter to your doctor requesting the requisition. This way it's not about the patient requesting a specific blood test, but one professional asking another.

- **Bring an advocate.** It's always helpful to bring someone with you to a doctor's appointment, whether it's your partner, a supportive friend, or family member. They can be there for emotional and moral support if you need it and can also listen closely — something you might not be able to do if you're upset during the appointment — and remind you to mention important details or think of questions you might not have considered. While it might seem strange to invite someone into the doctor's office with you, bringing an advocate to your appointment is your right.

- **Find a new doctor.** Also remember that your doctor is at your service. While it certainly might not feel that way given the power dynamic between patients and doctors, if you feel that your concerns aren't being taken seriously, you can find a new doctor if you have the ability to do so. I recognize that this is often easier said than done: smaller towns and rural areas might be lucky to have even one doctor. In the United States, insurance plans often have a list of approved doctors to choose from.

KEEP A COPY OF YOUR MEDICAL RECORDS

Your medical records are just that — *yours*. That means that you are entitled to see them and you are entitled to request a copy for your own records. I recommend that you always get a copy of test results and lab reports, and keep them in a safe place.

Get into the habit of requesting a copy of your test results or lab reports after your doctor's appointments. Some labs even allow you to access your test results through an online portal — and you may often be able to see the results before you see your doctor. If your doctor's office charges a small fee for photocopying, it is a worthwhile investment — getting your hands on your lab reports is the first step in advocating for yourself within the traditional medical system.

Having access to your own medical records means that your health and records are in your own hands, and it is the first step for advocating for yourself and taking control of your own health care. You will be able to look at how things change over time — an important aspect of preventative medicine, particularly when it comes to hormonal health. If you are consistently within lab ranges but notice that your levels are creeping higher or lower, depending on the hormone or nutrient in question, that can be a signal that something is changing and it may only be a matter of time before symptoms start showing up (if they haven't already). Having a copy of your own lab reports and blood tests can also help you look for errors — they happen, frequently — and certainly last but not least, it allows you to share the results with alternative practitioners that may not have the same access to test and lab results that your doctor will.

UNDERSTANDING YOUR TEST RESULTS

You don't have to have a medical degree to understand your test results. Some basic knowledge about what the tests are and how to understand lab ranges is all that you need.

Lab Ranges

When your doctor orders a blood test, they use what's called "lab ranges" to interpret the results. That's simply the range of what is considered to be healthy for that particular hormone or nutrient in the blood. When the results fall outside of that range, this indicates to your doctor that something is out of balance.

Lab ranges are a tool that your doctor uses to diagnose disease. It's the range your blood levels need to be at in order for you to function.

When it comes to hormonal health and nutrients in your blood levels, there is a difference between lab ranges and optimal ranges. It's entirely possible that you might present a number of symptoms that suggest an issue or imbalance, and yet your lab ranges are coming back normal. For your doctor, this might be case closed because everything looks normal. But you're left still feeling like shit.

There's a difference between just being alive and thriving. There are the ranges you need to keep the lights on (these would be lab ranges) and the ranges you need to thrive (optimal ranges). It's entirely possible that you feel like shit — your energy is low, you're constipated, your period is irregular, and when it does show up it's with a vengeance. And yet your lab ranges come back normal.

Optimal ranges are what you need not just to keep the lights on — but to thrive, free of symptoms.

Here's another thing about lab ranges — what if your blood tests three years in a row showed that your levels were within lab range, but changing year after year, creeping higher or lower. Is that an indication that something is amiss? When your doctor is looking at your lab results it's entirely possible that they're not going to compare your most recent test with the last time you had a blood test, particularly if your tests came back within lab range.

However, changes in your blood tests over time are something to look at and an important indicator that something is out of balance — it's like the whisper before the yell of a full-blown disease or illness. So, take note and don't be afraid to flag it to your health care provider.

ALTERNATIVE HEALTH AND PARAMEDICAL PRACTITIONERS

In the absence of a medical establishment that takes women's pain, and in particular menstrual-related symptoms, seriously, a wide arrange of alternative health and paramedical practitioners have stepped up to the fill void. Naturopathic doctors, Traditional Chinese Medicine practitioners, nutritionists, and physical therapists can help you to uncover the root cause of ovulation disturbances or menstrual pain and devise a treatment plan to address your issues. While the average time of an appointment with a general practitioner or specialist is about ten minutes, when you see an alternative practitioner you will likely have more time to discuss your concerns, health history, and potential solutions.

Unfortunately, many of these practitioners are private, meaning that you'll need to pay out of pocket to see them, in addition to paying for any additional supplements, herbs, or foods that they recommend. Not everyone can afford to pay upfront for health care, and not all insurance plans, if you have insurance, cover these modalities either, or do so only up to a limited amount per calendar year. If cost is an issue, seek out colleges in the modality that you're interested in trying. Many schools and colleges have teaching clinics that offer free services or reduced rates. Other clinics may also offer a sliding scale to make services more affordable and accessible to all that need them.

Here are some of the paramedical professionals and treatments that can help you improve your period.

Naturopathy

Naturopathic doctors will take a detailed health history and guide you through diet and lifestyle changes to improve your periods. They may also recommend specific nutritional supplements or botanical medicines, such as herbs, to help support your hormones; or they may use acupuncture and other elements of Traditional Chinese Medicine in your treatment plan.

Traditional Chinese Medicine and Acupuncture

Menstrual cycles are vital to health in Traditional Chinese Medicine (TCM), which makes TCM practitioners well suited to help you. Acupuncture, herbs, and diet and lifestyle practices are all part of the TCM toolbox. A TCM practitioner will make a diagnosis based on a detailed health history and physical exam and will prescribe the best course of treatment based on their assessment.

Pelvic Floor Physiotherapy

A relatively new modality that is gaining popularity in North America, pelvic floor physiotherapy works on the muscles in and around the vagina, uterus, diaphragm, and pelvic floor. While it is best known for post-pregnancy related issues like incontinence, pelvic floor therapy can also relieve menstrual-related complaints such as cramps or heavy flow. Endometriosis patients may find pelvic floor physiotherapy to be helpful for relieving tightness and pain from scarring or adhesions.

Massage

Getting a massage in the days before or during your period doesn't just sound like a luxurious way to pamper yourself — it can also be helpful to reduce tension, depression, or anxiety or to relieve pain and cramping. Ancient techniques like Maya Abdominal Massage have been specifically developed to bring blood flow to the uterus and position the uterus for more efficient menstrual flow.

Aromatherapy

Essential oils smell great and may have healing properties to help balance hormones and relieve pain. Depending on the oil and why you are using it, they can be inhaled using a diffuser or applied topically. As essential oils gain mainstream popularity, it is more important than ever to ensure that you are purchasing your oils from high quality, trusted sources. Pricing can be indicative of the quality of the ingredients. It's also important to use any essential oils under a knowledgeable, trained professional.

Herbalists

If you're interested in using herbs to support your hormonal and menstrual health, make sure that you consult a knowledgeable and experienced expert who can recommend the proper combination of herbs in the right dose. Many naturopathic doctors are trained in herbal medicine and can recommend herbs. Just because they're plants doesn't mean they can't be dangerous, particularly if you are taking other prescription medications that are contraindicated to herbs. You might be prescribed herbs in capsules, tinctures, teas, or even as a vaginal steam.

Nutritionists

Food has a tremendous influence on our hormones, as you will read in the following chapters, and hormonal health is a central pillar in holistic and functional nutrition. Making changes to your diet can feel overwhelming and challenging. A qualified nutritionist can help you implement changes to your diet and lifestyle to support your menstrual health.

Fertility Awareness Educators

Learning how to chart your cycle from a qualified fertility awareness educator is a key component to becoming body literate, particularly if you are planning on using fertility awareness to achieve or avoid pregnancy. A qualified practitioner can help you learn how to chart your cycles and interpret the signs and signals expressed within your cycle. They may also be able to make recommendations on specific nutrition and lifestyle changes to implement to support your cycle and hormonal health. See the resources section of this book for finding a fertility awareness educator who can help you learn to chart.

CHAPTER 7

THE NUTRITION APPROACH TO PERIOD CARE

Despite everything that we know about medicine, many still believe that there is nothing we can do about our bad periods: that our fate, by being born into a female body, is pain and inconvenience.

Throughout my teen years, while I was sewing my own pads and making zines about toxic tampons, I was still experiencing menstrual cramps and heavy bleeding. In my twenties, as I bounced from one brand of hormonal contraception to another, it was migraines that kept me home from work — but more often than not I powered through it; on more than one occasion I lay down right on my office floor to try and breathe through the pain.

Nutrition school was the first place where it was ever presented to me that my period didn't have to be a curse. My ears perked up — for one, despite being on hormonal contraceptives, I still experienced symptoms before my bleed that were unpleasant, to say the least. And, even more importantly, the one thing that kept me on hormonal birth control, despite feeling that it no longer fit with my wish to live a more organic, natural life, was the terror that the heavy, erratic periods that I had known in my teen years and any time I had gone off the pill in the past would return — perhaps with a vengeance.

I was right to be concerned. Because hormonal contraception doesn't regulate your period at all, but instead replaces your natural hormones with synthetic ones, symptoms aren't relieved but simply masked. When you begin taking hormonal contraception before your cycle matures around age twenty, your cycle doesn't have a chance to sort itself out. So, it's going to have to do that later in life when you come off of hormonal contraception.

Even if you haven't recently transitioned off hormonal birth control, or have never taken it at all, easier, more manageable periods are possible.

Our hormones are very sensitive to stress and nutrition, which means that a high-stress lifestyle and poor diet are going to adversely effect our hormonal health and, ultimately, our periods. Stress suppresses ovulation, and we need to ovulate in order to get the benefits of progesterone. If we're not making enough progesterone, estrogen can skyrocket without the counterbalance of progesterone, which contributes to period problems. And in a bizarre twist, higher levels of estrogen lead to higher levels of cortisol, a hormone that regulates our stress response — which in turn is going to affect our ability to ovulate.

And so, the cycle goes on and on.

The good news, however, is that food and lifestyle changes to reduce or manage stress can have a positive effect on our hormonal health and menstrual experience.

Looking at the evidence, there's an overwhelming case that the food we eat — or don't eat — has a profound effect on our hormones and therefore our menstrual health. PMS is linked to several deficiencies of vitamins and minerals, food allergies, and the body's ability to metabolize carbohydrates and essential fatty acids. Inflammation, a term that we're hearing about more and more in medical news, can contribute to pain, including menstrual cramps and breast tenderness, and is directly correlated with the food that we eat.

As such, it makes sense that a change in what we eat can have a positive effect on our day-to-day menstrual experience.

Our hormones respond well to nutrition and lifestyle changes — exercise, rest, relaxation, and perhaps most importantly, pleasure.

I can't think of a better way to counteract the stress of modern life then to focus on bringing more pleasure into our every day. We aren't often encouraged to do things just because they make us feel good or because we simply like them. So much of our pleasure is justified as "guilty" — from trashy novels to a daily square of dark chocolate. Rather than focusing on "stress management," I coach my clients to seek pleasure — even small acts of pleasure will chill us out, helping to balance our hormones and have a better period.

That means that making some changes to what we eat, how we move, and the thoughts that we think can have a positive impact on our hormonal health — and in turn, our menstrual cycles. We can manage some of the inflammation in our bodies through diet and lifestyle, which can help improve our period experience, promote ovulatory health, and keep our hormones humming along nicely.

On the most basic level, what we eat has a profound effect on our hormones because our hormones are made of what we eat. Changing the ingredients we use will change the final product. On a more complex level, our liver, a part of our digestive system, also plays a key role in hormone production. Hormones like insulin and cortisol are involved in our blood sugar response, and as we now know, no hormone is an island — they are all tightly regulated and balanced together. When one is out of sync, so goes the chain reaction down the line — eventually affecting your menstrual cycle.

Now, before we go on, it's time for some real talk. Be wary of diet culture masquerading as lifestyle changes to improve your health or cure disease.

I know from my own personal experience and the experience of my clients that what we eat, how we move, and the thoughts that we think absolutely have an impact — either positive or negative — on both the health of our menstrual cycles and overall health.

While you'll find nutritional guidelines and lots of information about how food affects your hormonal health and periods in this book, what you're not going to find is a highly prescriptive diet plan. In my view, true body literacy goes beyond menstrual cycles and hormonal health and extends all the way to what and how we eat.

Part of tuning in to your body, learning to tune in to its signals and cues, is learning how to eat intuitively. That means listening to your hunger cues, stopping when you've had enough, and eating from a place of self-care and compassion, rather than self-control.

We live in a diet culture that has a tight grip on all of us. Our society is obsessed with weight, shape, and size, prioritizing thinness and achieving a specific standard of beauty over health and wellness. Even as dieting trends shift towards a focus on "clean eating" or making "lifestyle changes," make no mistake — it's just a rebrand of the same old shit: dieting.

So if you make changes to what you eat as a way to improve your hormonal health, beware of getting too hung up on the rules. The guidelines that I offer in these pages are just that — guidelines.

My nutrition philosophy isn't centred around which foods are good or "clean" and which are bad and to be avoided at all costs. Nutrition is a spectrum of foods that offer more or less nutrition. That's it. I'm willing to bet that it's not breaking news to anyone living on this side of the planet that vegetables are nutritious and promote good health, while packaged, processed foods that are loaded with salt, sugar, and low-quality fats like cottonseed oil aren't.

You're a grown-up and you can eat what you want, when you want. After all, isn't that the beauty of being an adult? But I'm willing to bet that you also know the difference between how you feel when you've started your day with a sausage and egg McGriddle, two hash browns, and a French vanilla soy latte with extra syrup and when you've had a bowl of steel-cut oats topped with fresh fruit and nuts.

When you're tuned in to your body, you can listen to what it truly needs, at that moment, to fuel your life. What you do most of the time matters more than once in a while. So if most of the time what you need to start the day is the bowl of steel-cut oats, it doesn't matter if every so often that McGriddle is well and truly calling to you.

So much of improving your period experience is tied to pleasure and joy — more on that later — but pleasure and joy includes what you eat. A recent study showed that even a "perfect" diet made up of the most nutritious foods means nothing when you're stressed out — the effects of the stress will negate the nutrition in the food. Good news for your period, since stress can have an impact on that too.[1]

I believe pleasure should always be at the forefront of your food-related decision making. At the same time, nutrition is a long game. So, while your food should always taste good, sometimes the pleasure you take is the immediate gratification of an ooey, gooey fudgy brownie, and sometimes it's the pleasure of not feeling bloated in your afternoon meetings or doubled over with menstrual cramps the next time your period rolls around.

My last caveat before we get into nutrition for a better period is this: sometimes, no amount of kale or green juice is going to cure you. Food can be medicine, but it's not a panacea — if you're suffering from a serious disease that affects your menstrual cycle like endometriosis or adenomyosis, a diet change might help you manage your symptoms, but at the end of the day, it's not going to cure your disease.

Even so, I firmly believe that a change to nutrition and lifestyle factors like exercise and choosing natural, organic menstrual products should be the first line of defence when it comes to improving your menstrual experience.

In this section we'll discuss a holistic approach to supporting your hormonal health through nutrition and lifestyle changes.

GENERAL NUTRITIONAL GUIDELINES FOR HORMONAL HEALTH AND BETTER PERIODS

Let's start with some general guidelines that can improve the way anyone who gets a period (and likely even those that do not!) feels at any part of their cycle.

Eat What Makes You Feel Good

Recall my food philosophy: there are no good and bad foods, only food that is more or less nutritious. You don't need a nutrition degree to understand that the food that is more nutritious is going to make you feel well — that's stuff like vegetables, whole grains, and water. In turn, that general well-being will improve your period experience.

The key here is eating what makes you feel good. While there are some universal truths when it comes to nutrition — eating nothing but brownies will likely make you feel unwell while a varied, whole foods diet will likely make you feel vibrant — there is a lot of grey area in between, and that's where the experimentation comes in.

Bioindividuality ensures that each of us is made a little bit differently, and we all need something a little bit different in order to feel well. Our health history, genetics, and other factors such as the environment we grew up in and where we currently live all influence how we absorb and metabolize nutrients. There is no perfect diet that works for everyone, only the perfect diet for you, for right now. For example, there are a lot of people out there who thrive on a grain-free diet. And there are a lot of people out there who don't — myself included. I need some grains in my diet to really feel at my best, something that I've learned by experimenting over the years.

This isn't about experimenting with fad diets — it's about finding what makes you feel at your best and improves your period experience.

When I see clients, I ask them what foods they know they are sensitive to or find that make them feel unwell. To date, not a single client with hasn't listed at least one food that they just know doesn't make them feel great. What that food is, and how it makes them feel, varies from person to person. For some, it's a stomach ache or digestive upset immediately following eating dairy products. Others find that gluten triggers headaches or migraines, causes skin rashes, or changes their mood.

When it comes to eating what makes you feel good, simply removing the foods from your diet that you know or suspect don't make you feel great is always a good place to start.

If you don't know whether foods might be making you feel unwell, there are a few ways to investigate. I recommend starting with simple practices like taking a deep breath and tuning in to your body after you've eaten, or keeping a food and symptom journal, as these practices will not only help you identify any food sensitivities or intolerances, but also promote body literacy.

Here are a few ways you can start to understand how the foods that you eat are making you feel:

Check In After You Eat

The breathing exercises outlined in the previous chapter to help you get in tune with your body can also help you get in touch with how certain foods make you feel. Take a moment to check in and see how you feel when you put your fork down after a meal; then after thirty minutes; and again an hour or two later. If you're immediately feeling like you're bloated, your skin is itchy, your stomach hurts, or you have diarrhea (or all of the above), those are signs that you need to get a certain food out of your diet and start working on supporting your digestion. Food should leave you feeling satisfied and energized, not sluggish or uncomfortable — these are signs that what, or how, you're eating might be making you feel less than amazing.

Keep a Food and Symptom Journal

Connect specific foods to any symptoms that you might be experiencing. It really is as simple as jotting down what you've eaten alongside how you're feeling. You can use a paper journal, a note on your phone, or an app for tracking food and/or symptoms. Once you've been keeping track for even a short time you might notice that certain foods trigger adverse symptoms — for example, headaches, skin conditions, or digestive problems, although any unpleasant feeling can be tracked. The next step is to eliminate those foods and see what happens. While you eliminate any potentially offending foods, keep tracking what you eat alongside your symptoms. Aligning your food and symptom journal with your menstrual cycle charts can also help to identify any potential cycle-related or hormonal links.

Test for Food Sensitivities and Intolerances

Many naturopathic doctors, nutritionists, and functional medical specialists offer food sensitivity and intolerance tests through third-party labs. Depending on the company, tests use hair or blood samples to test the body's antibodies to foods.

I generally do not recommend this kind of testing to my clients because it's not uncommon for someone to get results that show they are sensitive to dozens, sometimes even hundreds, of different foods. They're often overwhelmed and stressed out, wondering what the heck they can eat. I much prefer an intuitive, observational approach like the food and symptom journal I explained above. I feel this will give you a more accurate picture while also encouraging you to really get to know your own body and how it reacts to specific foods rather than simply relying on a list. After all, the whole point is body literacy, right?

Try an Elimination and Challenge Diet

Completely eliminating common allergens is another way to determine food sensitivities or intolerances. You remove all common allergens (eggs, soy, dairy, wheat, and gluten) and inflammatory foods (sugar and processed foods) from your diet for a set period of time, usually a minimum of twenty-one days, and then introduce them one by one, closely monitoring whether any symptoms return.

While they may help you to determine food sensitivities, elimination diets can be challenging, possibly even harmful because they are so restrictive. I recommend trying an elimination diet only under the supervision of a nutritionist or other qualified practitioner who can help you appropriately reintroduce foods. After twenty-one or more days without pizza or whatever other foods you love but had to cut out, it's easy to binge. However, that can undo all your hard work, since eating more than one food you eliminated at the same time will make it impossible to know which foods caused your symptoms to return.

Get Tested for True Allergies

Your medical doctor or specialist can perform testing through blood tests or skin pricks to identify food allergies or diseases such as celiac, a true allergy to gluten.

Keep Your Blood Sugar Balanced

When it comes to hormonal and menstrual cycle health, blood sugar balance is one of the most important factors. It can also prevent other diseases like heart disease, Type II diabetes, and cancer.

The body process that helps to regulate the sugar levels in your bloodstream and transport sugar (as energy) into the cells is carried out by — you guessed it — hormones. Remember that hormones work together like an orchestra in your body; when one is out of balance it can throw off the whole band. If you're constantly riding the wave of blood sugar spikes and crashes, that's going to affect your insulin, cortisol, and adrenaline levels— all hormones — which will eventually have a downstream effect on your menstrual cycles.

Here's how the hormones that regulate your blood sugar work:

- **Insulin.** Made by the pancreas, insulin metabolizes fats and carbohydrates. It helps the liver and fat tissue convert glucose to glycogen, stored energy. Too much insulin will block the body's use of glycogen, converting it to fat.
- **Adrenaline.** Also known as epinephrine, it is critical to our short-term, acute stress response and it can be addictive. If you love the rush of a roller coaster or bungee jumping, that's adrenaline. This hormone kicks us in to high gear to run from a bear or make it through a short-term period of stress.
- **Cortisol.** Produced by the adrenal glands, cortisol responds to stress and helps to restore balance after a rush of adrenaline. It's also manufactured along the same metabolic pathways as progesterone — that means that if your body is busy making cortisol, it won't be making progesterone. Chronic stress and poor diet can elevate our cortisol secretions over time, which can have long-term effects, not the least of which is hormonal imbalance and menstrual disturbances, as well as increased inflammation and decreased immunity.

How Blood Sugar Regulates

Your blood sugar level is a measure of how much glucose is circulating in your blood. When we eat carbohydrates, which are converted to sugars, your body secretes insulin to convert it to energy. Sugar and refined carbohydrates — think fruit juice, baked goods or any type of "white foods" like bread, rice, or pasta — are easy to break down, and the resulting sugar rushes into your bloodstream, spiking your insulin levels as your body tries to use the onslaught of energy. Stimulants like alcohol, caffeine, and tobacco also affect your blood sugar balance.

Eventually your blood sugar crashes, which triggers a release of adrenaline to make sure that you don't hit the floor. If you've ever felt "hangry," that's adrenaline talking; you might feel anxious, irritable, shaky, or hyperalert. Adrenaline keeps your blood sugar up and then cortisol comes in to restore the balance.

Here's an example of how your blood sugar works in action. You wake up in the morning and your blood sugar levels are naturally low because you haven't eaten all night long. But you can barely get your bum out of bed, you're so tired and sluggish. So, the first thing you do is pour yourself a big mug of coffee to get your day started. The caffeine in the coffee revs your engine (that is, spikes your blood sugar) and you've now got the energy to get yourself out the door. On your way to work you stop to grab a chocolate croissant — maybe another coffee — and call it breakfast. Insulin kicks in to convert the sugar to energy and you're riding that sugar high. But by mid-morning you're starting to crash. Adrenaline kicks in to keep you going until you can find something to get your blood sugar levels back up again; you're likely craving more sugar because your body is going to look for the fastest source of energy that it can find — refined carbohydrates, perhaps in the form of a sugary drink or baked good. Once your blood sugar levels are back up, cortisol is released to restore the balance of the adrenaline.

And on it goes for the rest of the day until it's time for bed. Only when you hit the pillow you're dead tired, but still wide awake — *tired but wired*.

The take-home message here isn't that you should never eat a treat again — what you do most of the time matters more than what you do once in a while. And what you can do *most of the time* is avoid sugar spikes and crashes by balancing your blood sugar throughout the day.

Keeping your blood sugar balanced isn't difficult; it just means you need to pay a little attention to how you're assembling your meals or snacks. Here are some blood-balancing guidelines:

- **Protein and fat.** Protein and fat, as well as fibre, slow down digestion and create a slower, more sustained release of energy into the bloodstream. Combine a little protein and fat with your carbohydrates for every meal or snack. It will also likely keep you satisfied for longer, so you won't be hungry again so soon.

- **Whole grains and complex carbohydrates.** Complex carbohydrates are longer chain sugars that take longer to be digested. These include green leafy vegetables, starchy veggies like potatoes and sweet potatoes, beans, lentils, and whole grains. These types of carbohydrates score lower on the glycemic index, which means they are digested more slowly and give you sustained energy instead of the blood sugar spikes you'll get from sugar (of all kinds) and refined flours. Choose whole grains like brown rice, quinoa, or oats, and whole grain bread when you are itching for some toast.

THE HEALTHY SUGAR MYTH

Once you know the detrimental effects of too much sugar, the obvious next question is, "Okay, so what's a healthy form of sugar?"

It's a legitimate question and one that I get asked all the time; after all, who doesn't want a little sweetness in their lives?

Well … when it comes to sugar, the answer isn't as simple as what's "healthy" and what's not. Sweeteners like honey or maple syrup are often labelled as "natural" or even "healthy," but at the end of the day they are still forms of sugar, which means they have the same effect on your blood sugar, and therefore your hormones, menstrual cycle, and overall health.

So what is the difference between "refined" and "natural" sweeteners?

When most people talk about sugar they are referring to the highly refined white sugar that you find in the sugar bowl, candy, and desserts. This sugar has been highly processed and stripped of any fibre or nutrition, leaving you with pure carbohydrates. On the Glycemic Index white sugar scores 100. Brown sugar, cane sugar, and specialty sugars like turbinado, demerara, or sucanat are still all refined sugar — just processed a little differently! However, they have been cleverly marketed to appear as "healthy" alternatives.

The sweeteners often considered to be "natural" are things like maple syrup, honey, coconut sugar, or brown rice syrup, which all fall around 50 or less on the Glycemic Index. They are not as highly refined as white sugar and therefore still contain some vitamins or minerals, as well as some fibre to help slow the absorption in your body. That's why they score lower on the Glycemic Index.

However, let's be real — I wouldn't consider any natural sweetener to be a good source of nutrients. Anything you can find in a sweetener you can find in a vegetable or fruit. Raw honey does contain a host of unique enzymes, phytonutrients, and other nutritional benefits not found elsewhere, but it's still a sugar and doesn't get a free pass to be consumed all the time!

I am the last person who would ever tell you that you should have absolutely no sweets in your life; my point is, any natural sweetener is still a sugar and should be treated as such. When I'm baking in my own kitchen I always reach for maple syrup or coconut sugar, but I also realize that you can still have too much of a good thing; too many naturally sweetened cookies are still too many cookies.

THE GLYCEMIC INDEX

The Glycemic Index is a system for ranking foods based on the effects they have on blood sugar levels. The Index is ranked from 0 to 100, with pure glucose scoring 100. Using the Glycemic Index is a great way to start understanding how foods affect your blood sugar. However, it's not a perfect system — it's not unusual to find some whole foods scoring higher on the Glycemic Index than some processed, packaged, or "junk" foods. Keep in mind that this measure is only looking at how foods affect your blood sugar and doesn't take any other nutrition factors into account.

SUPPORTING YOUR DIGESTION

What does your digestion have to do with your period? Well, a lot actually.

For starters, excess hormones like estrogen exit through, shall we say, the back door. If you're not passing a bowel movement regularly — and efficiently, because not every poop is created equal — excess hormones, like estrogen, are hanging around in your lower intestine and will be reabsorbed into the bloodstream, where they will continue to act on hormone receptors. This is what can lead to estrogen dominance.

> **A NOTE ABOUT ORGANIC SWEETENERS**
> The difference between regular and organic sugar doesn't have anything to do with nutrition or how it's used by your body. Anything that has been certified as organic has been grown and/or processed without synthetic pesticides, fertilizers, or other additives.

Higher levels of estrogen and the age of the estrogen in your system can be linked to myriad period symptoms — from PMS to low progesterone. During the follicular phase of your cycle, estrogen is responsible for thickening the uterine lining; the more estrogen you have, the thicker the endometrium might grow. When there is more lining to shed, your periods are longer, heavier, and can be accompanied by clots and more painful cramps because the uterus works harder to shed the endometrium. The age of the estrogen also has an effect on your menstrual experience.

To keep those hormones moving, make sure you're going to the bathroom regularly and efficiently. Drink enough water; get enough good sources of both soluble and insoluble fibre in your diet from leafy green vegetables, whole grains, and seeds like flax and chia. Eat fermented foods like sauerkraut, kimchi, or yogurt, and drink low-sugar kombucha. Dairy products and highly processed foods can clog the drain, so avoid them.

The other link between your digestion and your menstrual cycle is through your liver, which is part of your digestive system. This hard-working organ has more than five hundred jobs to do! It's responsible for detoxification and bile production, and also plays a role in hormone metabolization.

If your liver is overworked trying to detox from too much wine and polluted air, hormone production may take a backseat. When your body is busy just trying to keep the lights on — i.e., just trying to keep you upright and breathing — it's not going to be focused on reproduction. As a result, your hormones may become imbalanced, causing irregular periods, amenorrhea, or unpleasant PMS symptoms.

Detoxification isn't something that you do every once in a while; your liver is constantly working to detoxify so it needs some support, daily. I don't believe in "detoxing to re-tox" — the harsh detox done once a year that's designed as a quick fix to atone for the sins of poor nutrition choices and too much alcohol, caffeine, tobacco, or other stimulants. This approach is short-sighted and isn't going to do much to support your body long-term, never mind have any effect on your hormonal health.

Instead, give your liver some daily love by easing your toxic load:

- Minimize the alcohol you consume.
- Don't smoke.
- Eliminate toxicants in your home that are found in cleaning and personal care products.
- Use a high-quality air filter in your home.
- Choose organic foods and personal care products if and when you can.
- Include foods that support your liver function in your diet, including beets and bitter, leafy greens.
- Install a water filter in your shower and kitchen sink.

Organic and natural products aren't always accessible to everyone, either because they aren't available or come at a steep premium, so prioritize them when and where you can. We're not aiming for perfection or to be 100 percent toxin-free (although, ideally, we wouldn't have to be making these types of choices), simply to make manageable changes whenever possible.

KEEPING YOUR THYROID HEALTHY

Although your thyroid, a butterfly-shaped gland located at the base of your throat, and the hormones that it secretes, aren't directly implicated in your menstrual cycle, the two are tightly interconnected. Issues related to the thyroid commonly show up in menstrual cycle charts, and many menstrual disturbances are common symptoms of an underactive thyroid.

Thyroid hormones act on every single cell in your body. The thyroid is required for the manufacturing of proteins and stimulates calorie burn. In other words, we need our thyroid to work properly in order for the rest of our bodies to function.

An underactive thyroid, known as hypothyroidism, can have an effect on your menstrual cycle in many ways. It can contribute to heavy bleeding, causes anovulation (which lowers progesterone), impairs the metabolism of estrogen, and stimulates prolactin (which suppresses ovulation and worsens insulin resistance, a factor in PCOS). Irregular periods, heavy periods, and infertility may all be signs of an underactive thyroid.

When it comes to testing, the standard thyroid test looks at thyroid-stimulating hormone (TSH). An underactive thyroid will actually show up as *higher* levels of TSH on lab results. Criteria vary, and a result of anywhere between 3 mIU/L and 5 mIU/L can classify as an underactive thyroid. Standard tests generally look only at TSH but there are other tests that measure thyroid hormones, including thyroid peroxidase (TPO), an enzyme that helps to synthesize TSH, thyroid antibodies, and free T3 and T4. If you or your health care provider suspect an issue with your thyroid, particularly in PCOS, or if the autoimmune disorder Hashimoto's is suspected, ensure that you're not being tested just for TSH.

Because all of our hormones work together, recommendations for supporting your menstrual cycle hormones will also be beneficial for your thyroid health. Increasing the amount of iodine-rich foods like sea salt, sea vegetables, and seafood, as well as selenium, can be beneficial.

REDUCING YOUR INFLAMMATION

Inflammation has received a lot of attention in recent years, and for good reason. Scientists are discovering links between inflammation and many chronic diseases, as well as menstrual pain.

Pain and cramping before and during your period can be attributed to prostaglandins, which are hormone-like substances that are released as part of your body's pain and inflammatory response. They are also responsible for triggering the uterine contractions that allow the lining to be shed from your uterus. Studies have found that the more severe the cramps, the higher the levels of prostaglandins in a woman's body. The same is true for those of us suffering from conditions such as endometriosis.

Reducing the overall amount of inflammation in your body can have a positive effect on your period pain simply because you will have fewer prostaglandins in your body overall.

Focusing your diet on whole, unprocessed foods is the best way to start. Get rid of overly processed, packaged foods. Keep your blood sugar balanced, as prolonged secretions of cortisol can increase inflammation levels. Food that you are sensitive or allergic to can contribute to inflammation, so avoid anything that you know isn't going to make you feel absolutely amazing.

BEING MINDFUL OF HOW YOU EAT

Eating is one life's greatest pleasures and it should be treated as such: a pleasure. Luckily, pleasure is one of the keys to improving your period health — so the benefits of mindful eating are twofold: you'll get to enjoy your food more, and your menstrual health will benefit from that added pleasure. Downing a sandwich in the car or drinking a smoothie as you dash from one meeting to the next isn't my idea of pleasurable, and consuming food this way is going to catch up to you. How you eat impacts your digestion, which is a key factor in improving your hormonal and menstrual health.

Digestion begins even before you've put a single thing in your mouth. You know when you've got something that looks and smells incredible on the plate in front of you and your mouth starts to water? That's your body revving its digestive engine, getting ready to start the process of digestion. Even the act of preparing your food helps to get the digestive juices flowing.

Are you even chewing your food when you eat? There's a good chance you're not. If you need to push your food down with liquids, you're not chewing properly.

Not paying attention to the meal in front of us is another digestion killer — if you're watching TV or scrolling through Instagram, you're not thinking about eating. Not paying attention while you're eating can lead to over-eating, since you're not tuned in to your body's satiety cues.

So the next time you're hungry, treat yourself to a meal. Set aside at least twenty minutes and sit down at a real table, in a real chair; use a real plate and real cutlery. If you absolutely can't get away from your desk at lunchtime, at least move your chair over so that you're not directly in front of your computer. Thoroughly chew each bite until it's liquid, or close to it, putting your fork down after each bite. At the end of your meal, take a moment to check in and see how you feel.

Using food to support your hormonal and menstrual health isn't just about *what* you eat — *how* you eat is just as, if not more, important. Taking time out of your busy day to really focus on the pleasure of eating will help to improve digestion and tap into that "rest and digest" mode that is essential for lowering stress.

Now that we've covered the big "why's" for using nutrition to have a better period, we'll dive deeper into specific foods that help or hinder our hormonal health in the following chapter.

CHAPTER 8
FOODS FOR SUPPORTING HORMONAL HEALTH

As I listened to my instructors over the years in nutrition school, I noticed a pattern emerge: it didn't seem to matter whether we were talking about diets for diabetes, pregnancy, or periods — the common thread was simply to *eat real food*.

While it almost seems too simple, it really is that easy: focusing on eating fresh vegetables, fruits, whole grains, and a little good quality protein and fat, most of the time is going to have a profound effect on your periods, and your health in general.

The only diet advice you ever need comes from Michael Pollan, author of *In Defense of Food: An Eater's Manifesto*: "Eat food. Not too much. Mostly plants."

I'm going to go out on a limb here and guess that it's probably not news that eating vegetables is good for you. At the same time, I know that living a modern life — juggling work and life and family and other priorities — can make it seem daunting and overwhelming to follow even the simplest guidelines. The food industry's marketing messages are powerful and loud. Just as we've been sold period shame, we've also been led to believe that real, wholesome food is more expensive, difficult to prepare, and takes a long time.

If body literacy is an act of resistance, buying, cooking, and eating real food is too. It might take an investment in time and or energy at the get-go, but the long-term gains cannot be underestimated.

A note about calories: as a holistic nutritionist, I am generally more concerned about the nutritional value of the foods that you're eating versus counting calories. Not all calories are created equal! A hundred calories of almonds are not equal to a hundred calories of Oreo cookies — the almonds contain both the micro- and macro-nutrients that you need to function and build health, while the other doesn't. Getting hung up on how many calories you're eating is highly restrictive and can lead to disordered eating and eating disorders — and don't get me wrong, getting hung up on how many nutrients you're getting in a day does, too. The focus should be on eating a wide variety of foods with an intuitive approach — eating when you're hungry, stopping when you're full, and honouring your cravings.

That said, not getting enough calories or nutrition is a factor in many menstrual disorders, particularly amenorrhea or absent periods. If you're not getting enough calories to support your activity levels, or if you are eating sufficient calories, but the food that you're eating isn't giving you the nutrition that your body needs, it will be reflected in your hormones and menstrual cycle. Be sure that you're eating enough to sustain your activity levels and that you're eating whole foods most of the time.

If you struggle with an eating disorder or disordered eating and your period has stopped, please seek the attention of a qualified medical professional to treat your eating disorder before you attempt to repair your period.

Okay, are you ready? Here are the building blocks of a nutritious, health-promoting diet that will support your hormonal health through all phases of your life cycles, including pregnancy, breastfeeding, and well into menopause.

Plant-Based Foods

First and foremost, I advocate for a plant-based diet. Seriously, if you only implement one nutritional change from this entire book, let it be adding plants to your menu. Lots of them.

A diet that is rich in vegetables and other plants is high in fibre and anti-inflammatory properties, two things that are essential for supporting your menstrual cycle and improving your period experience. This doesn't necessarily mean being vegan or even vegetarian — although studies show that vegetarians have 15 to 20 percent lower estrogen levels in their blood[1] — it simply means that the majority of your diet is made up of plants: vegetables; fruits; whole grains; fats from plant-based sources such as olives, nuts, or coconuts; and plant proteins like beans, lentils, legumes, nuts, and seeds.

A quick rule of thumb for eating plant-based: is the majority of your plate made up of plants? If not, throw in a salad, a handful of raw vegetables like baby carrots or celery, or a green juice.

Vegetables

Fresh vegetables, particularly of the leafy green variety, are filled with micronutrients — the vitamins and minerals that our cells need to function. Menstrual cycle disturbances are closely linked with nutrient deficiencies. Plant foods also contain antioxidants, which we need to protect our cells from damage; and they are, of course, a great source of fibre.

Eat a wide variety of vegetables every day, both raw and cooked. Different-coloured vegetables contain different nutrients, so try to put as many colours on your plate as you can. In other words, eat the rainbow. Starchy vegetables like potatoes, sweet potatoes, carrots, and beets are a great source of carbohydrates to keep your energy levels up without the sugar rush of refined carbs from bread or sugar.

Whole Grains

Whole, intact grains are a terrific source of fibre as well as B vitamins — which we need to support hormonal health. And there are lots to choose from beyond brown rice! Stock your pantry with wild rice, quinoa, millet, oats, farro, buckwheat, wheat berries, and other hearty grains. Farro, spelt, and wheat berries contain wheat and are not gluten free. Some oats may contain gluten from cross-contamination in processing; look for certified gluten-free oats if you need to.

Fats

Contrary to the diet advice of the eighties, our bodies need fat. It's essential for our brain health, nervous system, and, you guessed it, our hormones. Fat also helps to slow down digestion and keeps you satiated for longer. The

---

MAKE GRAINS MORE DIGESTIBLE

If you find grains are hard to digest, soak them overnight with a splash of apple cider vinegar. This will help to break down the phytic acid, a compound found in plant seeds (that is, grains and beans) that makes them difficult to digest. You can also purchase sprouted varieties in many health food stores and most high-end grocery stores these days, although they are more expensive. Soaking them does the trick too!

best sources of fat are high-quality butter or ghee (clarified butter often used in South Asian cooking); avocados; extra virgin, cold-pressed oils, including coconut, olive, flax, and hemp; and raw nuts and seeds.

Protein

The amino acids found in protein are the building blocks of the cells that make up our bodies, including hormones. Protein helps to keep us more full for longer, and builds muscle. You might be surprised to learn that protein isn't only found in meat or other animal-based foods; many plant foods, and not just beans and legumes, also contain protein. When it comes to hormonal health, protein is essential, so this is one place where I do recommend a good quality supplement in the form of protein powder to make sure that you're getting not just enough, but optimal amounts for hormonal health. Look for unsweetened varieties made from whey (if you can handle dairy) or beef, or vegetarian sources of protein from pea protein or hemp. Many bulk food stores now sell protein powder so you can buy only what you need for a week or two at a time instead of a giant bodybuilder's tub.

Fruit

Just like your vegetables, fruit is a great source of vitamins and minerals, which again we can see from their brilliant colours. I believe that fruit is an essential part of our diets, but we need to be mindful of the fact that it does contain fructose, a type of sugar. Thankfully, nature also built in fibre to most fruits, which helps to slow down digestion and the release of sugar into our bloodstream. So, I recommend eating fruit in its whole form rather than, say, in fruit juice, which has been stripped of fibre and will affect your blood sugar levels. Pair your fruit with some fat and protein, like an apple with almond butter, for example, to slow down the sugar spike.

Fermented Foods

Yup, I'm putting fermented foods into their own food group. The microbiome in our body is made up of countless microbes — the good, and at times not-so-good, bacteria that we need to live. These bacteria aren't bad; in fact, they are essential to our health and wellness. Stress, inflammation, hormonal birth control, poor diet, and food allergies can all contribute to an imbalance of these microbes. If the bad bacteria outweigh the good, it can lead to all kinds of symptoms — from digestive upsets to hormonal imbalance. Given this, it's essential that we support and replenish our microbiome with probiotic fermented foods. Sauerkraut, kimchi, kombucha, miso, and yogurt are all great sources that are easy to make at home or are gaining mainstream popularity and are easier and easier to find in grocery and health food stores. But these aren't the only fermented foods out there — cultures around the world all have their own. Try them all until you find what you like! While they might take some getting used to, start with a small amount and work your way up — and try a wide variety. I recommend eating or drinking a quarter to a half cup of fermented foods daily. Be aware that they can also contribute to loose stools, so start with a small serving and work your way up to bowel tolerance.

Water

Staying hydrated is essential to every single cell in our body and is key for digestion, especially keeping things regular and moving along, which means your body is getting rid of excess hormone waste before it's reabsorbed into the bloodstream where it can wreak havoc on your periods. How much water you need varies greatly depending on your weight, activity level, the climate that you live in, the foods that you eat — many vegetables and fruits have a high-water content and contribute to your hydration — and how much alcohol and caffeine you consume, as both have a diuretic effect and can be dehydrating. A good rule of thumb is to watch the colour of your urine. It should be clear or pale yellow. Thick, cloudy urine can be a sign of dehydration, as can headaches. Drink water throughout the day, more on hot days or when you're doing intense workouts, and watch for signs of dehydration.

Treats

I'm calling it: treats are essential and deserve their own food group. Perhaps one of the best things about being a human is getting to eat for pleasure — and pleasure is such a key component to maintaining hormonal health. This means that there is definitely room for treats in a diet that supports your hormonal health and menstrual cycle. What you do most of the time matters more than what you do once in a while; some chocolate or a glass of wine — or maybe both — isn't going to be the undoing of your hormonal health. However, the quantity you consume within the context of your overall diet is something to consider. Listen to your cravings — are you really hungry for sweets or chips or is it something else that you're after? And listen to how these treats make you feel. Intuitive eating is a piece of body literacy.

FOODS THAT HINDER HORMONAL HEALTH

While I am a strong believer that there are no bad foods, there are a handful that are known to have an adverse effect on our hormones, which means they can mess with your menstrual cycles and your periods.

I've outlined these foods below, but here are a few caveats before we begin:

- Get to know how these foods affect *you*. We are all different, and what's most important is how specific foods make us feel and affect our own health and hormones.
- Figure out how much of these foods you're really eating — you might be eating more of certain ingredients than you think, especially if you're eating a lot of processed and packaged foods. Just because you're not drinking soy milk lattes or throwing tofu into your stir-fry every night doesn't mean you're not eating soy daily, for example. Read labels.
- Understand that reducing or cutting out specific foods likely doesn't mean forever.... Unless you have a known allergy, like celiac, you likely won't have to avoid a specific food for the rest of your life. There will always be times that call for just going for it — even if you know that you might not feel your best the next day (there is a reason why "When in Rome" is a saying). And that's a-okay. If I've said it once, I've said it a hundred times — what you do most of the time matters more than what you do once in a while. So, if you avoid cow's dairy on a regular basis, that doesn't mean you need to skip out on your family's once-a-year run to the old-timey diner for a banana split. Pleasure is an essential nutrient.

Below are the foods that are known to affect your hormones and that you may want to reduce or eliminate altogether, depending on your symptoms and how they affect you.

Soy

Soy has long been debated as both a friend and foe to hormonal health, largely because of the phytoestrogens it contains.

> ### WEEKEND WARRIOR SYNDROME
> Beware the weekend warrior syndrome — this is when someone avoids a food that they may be sensitive to throughout the week, only to go whole hog on the weekends. If you have a known food sensitivity or allergy, this type of eating pattern isn't going to help you improve your health and repair your hormones. If you're sensitive to a particular food, I recommend that you work with a qualified practitioner who can help you remove it from your diet and safely reintroduce it once symptoms have subsided to see if it is still causing concerns for your health.

Phytoestrogens are plant-derived compounds with both pros and cons.[2] They have been reported to have numerous health-promoting benefits, such as lowering your risk of cardiovascular disease, breast cancer, and symptoms related to menopause. At the same time, some phytoestrogens are also considered to be endocrine disruptors, which means that they can contribute to health issues, particularly PMS, ovarian cysts, and PCOS.

Unfortunately, the only answer I have to the question of whether or not you should eat soy is: it depends!

First of all, how much soy you're consuming is a big factor in whether or not it's health-promoting. While many Asian cultures regularly eat soy, they're doing so in small amounts each day. They're not eating soy yogurt and soy hot dogs, followed by soy ice cream or smoothies that have been stacked with soy protein.

Now, here's where it gets tricky when it comes to soy. You might think that you're not consuming a lot of (if any) soy because you don't eat tofu or drink soy milk. But if you take a look at just about any prepackaged or processed food label, you're likely to find some sort of soy product listed — soy protein isolate, soybean oil, soy lecithin. So, it turns out you might be eating more soy than you think.

Beyond phytoestrogens, soy is a contentious food because it is one of the most commonly genetically modified crops out there. As a cash crop, it's also often loaded with pesticides.

Here's where your body literacy comes in. How does soy make you feel? How much soy are you really consuming? Do you have a hormone or menstrual-related issue that is tied to estrogen dominance, like PMS or a heavy flow? How you answer these questions will determine whether or not you should be eating soy.

If you do eat soy, choosing soy products that are organic and sprouted, or better yet fermented like tempeh or miso, is the best way to ensure that you're getting the best quality form of soy.

Dairy

Telling someone that they need to cut down on or remove dairy from their diet is always a little heart-breaking, as I'm a certified cheese lover. However, the evidence is clear that dairy products, particularly those made from cow's milk, have an adverse effect on our hormonal health.

Milk and products made from milk — cheese, yogurt, butter, cream, ice cream — can have an effect on our hormonal health; particularly when it's cow's milk. Milk, whether it comes from a cow, sheep, goat, or even a human, is designed for babies and is full of the hormones that are needed to help stimulate the growth of said babies.

So, when you're ingesting milk, you're also ingesting those hormones, which is going to impact your hormone levels, and in turn your menstrual health. Limiting the amount of dairy that you consume and choosing sheep- or goat's-milk products over cow's milk can be beneficial to your hormones.

Dairy is also a common allergen and many people are sensitive to it, which means that on top of the endocrine-disrupting properties, you may also experience inflammation and irritation in your gut, contributing to internal stress and digestive issues.

Sugar

Sugar — in all its forms, even the supposed "healthy" versions — has an effect on your menstrual health because your blood sugar response, the function that helps usher energy from the bloodstreams into the cells, is regulated by hormones. Constantly riding blood sugar spikes and crashes can put us into a state of chronic stress. Cortisol, a stress hormone, is manufactured along the same pathways as progesterone, the key hormone of our menstrual cycles. There is also a link between PCOS and insulin resistance.

Gluten

There was a time, not that long ago, when a gluten-free diet was all the rage. It sparked a lot of news headlines and debate about whether or not we all needed to be gluten free. The truth is that no, we probably don't all need to be gluten free. Food marketers quickly caught on to the buzz attached to the gluten-free craze, however, and a walk down a supermarket aisle reveals no shortage of gluten-free foods. Suddenly everything from bags of chips to ice cream was now being touted as gluten free. But here's the thing — just because something is gluten free doesn't mean that it promotes health. Junk food can be gluten free.

There are many people out there who do need to avoid gluten because of a true allergy or celiac disease. And then there are those people who don't have celiac, but still do better on a gluten-free diet — this is known as non-celiac gluten sensitivity.

There appears to be a link between non-celiac gluten-sensitivity and infertility.[3] Thus, one may also conclude it's possible that there's a link between gluten sensitivity and hormonal health. Celiac disease and gluten intolerance interrupt your hormonal health by increasing inflammation, contributing to nutritional deficiencies, and disrupting the microbiome in your gut and vagina. One study found that a gluten-free diet reduced endometriosis-related pain symptoms in 75 percent of participants.[4]

These are compelling arguments for reducing or avoiding gluten if you're experiencing painful periods or hormonal imbalances — going gluten-free might just be a key component to having a better period experience. However, as I mentioned above, beware the gluten-free junk-food diet. Gluten-free doesn't automatically mean healthy. Conversely, if what you eat most of the time is whole and plant-based foods, you will naturally be reducing the amount of gluten in your diet. Vegetables, fruits, beans, legumes, and whole grains — with the exception of wheat and some oats that may have been contaminated — are all naturally gluten-free and hormonal-health supporting.

When it comes to gluten, my advice, like everything else in this book, is to get to know what works for you. If you know that gluten immediately makes you feel like garbage, take it out — although also keep in mind that we often consume gluten alongside other inflammatory, common allergens like dairy and sugar in the form of pizza or cookies. So, was it really the gluten or was it something else that was affecting you? Keeping a food journal and eliminating/challenging foods one at a time will help you figure it out and find the best diet for you and your hormonal health.

If you do suspect that you have a true gluten allergy or celiac disease, note that you will need to have consumed gluten for at least six weeks prior to your blood test — the only way for the blood test to be accurate is for the antibodies to be present in your bloodstream. No gluten, no antibodies.

RESTRICTIVE DIETS/LIFESTYLES

Living in the diet-obsessed culture that we do, it's difficult to open a magazine, go online, or even watch the evening news without some mention of one diet or another. But here's the deal with diets: I'm not into them. Not at all, including the diets designed to "optimize" your menstrual cycles.

Labels should be saved for your jeans or a can of beans, not what or how you eat. I don't believe that there is one diet or one approach to eating that works for everyone, all the time. What and how much you need to feel your best is going to change from day to day, cycle to cycle, year to year. Finding the perfect diet for you isn't about following a meal plan or program; it's about experimentation to find what's best for you, as we discussed in the previous pages.

Here I have included some food for thought on some of the popular diets that you're likely to brush up against.

Going Vegetarian or Vegan

Choosing whether or not to eat meat is a complex decision. Vegetarianism sits at the intersection of health, food, the environment, politics, and morality. As a nutritionist, I don't believe in prescriptive diets, and that includes strictly adhering to a vegan or a vegetarian diet.

When it comes to hormonal health, this is one of those things that seems to be polarizing. For every Instagram influencer out there claiming that a paleo diet fixed her periods, you'll find another that had success with an entirely plant-based vegan diet.

Studies have shown that vegetarians have lower levels of estrogen in their bloodstreams than omnivores. Meat-eaters tend to eat less fibre than vegetarians or vegans, which is another contributing factor to hormonal health and general well-being.

So what to do? I encourage you to experiment and figure out what's right for you. How much, if any, meat do you need to feel your best? What aligns with your values? Also recognize that the answers to those questions might change depending on where you are in your cycle — many people crave animal protein, particularly red meat, when they are bleeding, perhaps because of the amount of iron that they are losing during their flow, or the seasons, or where you are in your life.

If you ultimately decide that a vegan or vegetarian diet is what best aligns with your politics and values, it's important not to rely on overly processed soy, imitation meat products, or other vegetarian convenience foods. They might not be made of animal protein, but they can still be inflammatory and wreak havoc on your gut health. Put these types of foods in the "treat" category.

Vegan and vegetarian diets should also be supplemented with vitamins and minerals, including B complex vitamins, zinc, and omega-3 fatty acids.

Going Paleo or Keto

If nutrition is a spectrum, then certainly it seems that being vegan is at one end and paleo or keto diets are at the other end. Both are based on low- to no-carbohydrate intake, instead focusing on protein and fat for energy. Both of these diets have received a lot of attention, particularly on social media, for being a cure-all for hormone-related issues.

Lara Briden, a naturopathic doctor, writes that while these types of very low carbohydrate diets seem to have an initial period of effectiveness, after a period of six months or so they can actually contribute to hormonal imbalances.

Remember that carbohydrates are our body's main source of energy, and not getting enough energy has been associated with amenorrhea, which means that it can disrupt our hormones. For this reason, I hesitate to recommend a very low carb diet for everyone.

Weight Loss Diets

Any type of restrictive diet that promises weight loss falls into this category. And let me tell you this: it's all bullshit. It doesn't matter if it's South Beach or a clean eating "lifestyle change" or any other diet that promises to help you shed pounds — stay far, far away. Contrary to popular health advice, you don't have to be skinny to be healthy. And like period shame or taboo, diet culture is a tool of the patriarchy designed to keep women occupied with their bodies instead of, I don't know, becoming bilingual or climbing a mountain or just being the incredible, awesome person that you are. If you struggle with breaking out of restrictive diet patterns, I encourage you to seek help from an experienced mental health professional and intuitive eating nutritionist or food therapist who can help you reclaim the joy of food.

IS EATING ORGANIC IMPORTANT?

Here's another hotly debated nutrition topic: whether or not you need to be eating organic. And as with the question of whether or not you need to be vegetarian, the answer is complex. So, let's break down the facts.

Organic food has been grown and processed without any synthetic pesticides, fertilizers, or other additives. It's used by your body in the same way as non-organic foods, and it contains all the same types of nutrients that non-organic foods do. Some studies have shown that organic food isn't necessarily better for you from a nutritional standpoint. Many holistic health practitioners or wellness advocates disagree, believing that organic foods contain more nutrients by virtue of the quality of the soil that it is grown in.

That said, the pesticides, fertilizers, and other stuff found in conventionally grown produce and food have been shown to be harmful to our health. Many are known carcinogens, meaning that they can cause cancer. They can also be endocrine disruptors, which we know means that they will interfere with our hormones, and thus have an adverse effect on our menstrual health and fertility. Studies suggest that endocrine disrupting chemicals affect both male and female fertility; they may impair hormone function and sperm production and may inhibit ovulation and reduce egg quality. They may also exacerbate PCOS and endometriosis.[5]

Considering the evidence, the choice seems obvious — there are clear benefits for eating organic foods. If you're looking to improve your hormonal health and have a better period, organic foods are a great choice. However, the reality is that organic foods and other products, such as makeup or personal care products, are more expensive and not always available. At the end of the day, eating fresh produce is more important than eating fresh *organic* produce.

In a perfect world we wouldn't need to make this kind of choice, but our world is far from perfect. We're exposed to countless harmful toxins in our day-to day-lives, not just from the foods we eat, but from the water we drink, the air we breathe, the clothes we wear, and the products we use to clean ourselves and our homes. The goal isn't to be 100 percent organic all of the time — because it would be just about impossible — but rather to lower your toxic load by prioritizing organic food and other products in key areas that will have the most impact.

Below are a few ways to make the switch without blowing the bank.

Avoid the Dirty Dozen™

The Environmental Working Group (EWG) publishes an annual Shoppers Guide to Pesticides in Produce™ guide. The guide outlines the "Dirty Dozen," those foods that rank highest in terms of pesticide residue and the crops that are typically grown with genetically modified seeds. The guide also includes the "Clean 15" — foods that are on the other end of the spectrum and typically rank low in terms of pesticide residue.[6] Prioritize buying organic for those fruits and veggies that make the Dirty Dozen™ List.

Another way to prioritize which foods to buy organic is to consider which produce you peel and which fruits or veggies have edible skin. Although pesticides and chemicals can be absorbed through the peel or skin into the flesh, they're less concentrated in the flesh. For example, avocados and melons have thick skins that we peel and discard, while we generally eat the skin on an apple or pear and eat berries whole.

Eat Locally and with the Seasons

In general, the further food has to travel to make it to the consumer the more pesticides it's treated with to keep it fresh on the long journey. And to make sure it's ripe — not overripe — upon arrival, these foods are picked before they are ready and allowed to "ripen on the truck," often with the help of chemicals. Buying your food from farmers' markets and local sources can often mean lower exposure to pesticides, even if it's not certified organic. Organic certification is a costly and lengthy process that many small farms can't afford to pursue, even if they are growing according to organic practices. Shopping at a farmers' market means you can get to know the people behind your food and how it's grown, even if it doesn't have an official seal or sticker.

Subscribe to a CSA or Produce Delivery

Community Supported Agriculture (CSA) and produce deliveries cut out the middle men and bring organic produce right to the consumer — that is, your doorstep or a designated drop-off point in your neighbourhood, which means that you're not paying the retail mark-up that you would at the grocery store or health food store.

Avoid Organic Junk Food

A bag of organic cheese puffs is still a bag of cheese puffs; the ingredients have just been grown without pesticides. Don't fall for the health halo of organic junk food, or other labels like "natural" or "gluten-free," for that matter. This can make a big difference in saving money. Skip the premium mark-up on organic chips and divert those funds to your veggie budget instead!

Ultimately, the advice that I give to my clients is to first focus on eating plants. Then once you find your flow, you can fit in local and organic foods where you can.

NUTRITIONAL DEFICIENCIES AND YOUR MENSTRUAL CYCLE

Micronutrients like vitamins and minerals are the building blocks of our cells and help our bodies function. Nutrient deficiencies are one of the things that can show up in your menstrual charts, and are linked with PMS, irregular periods, and menstrual-related disorders like endometriosis or PCOS.

A key thing to remember when it comes to your diet: it's best to focus on the big picture and not get hung up on specific micronutrients. That means focusing on eating a wide variety of foods from each food group rather than nitpicking about which berries have the highest vitamin C content. Eating a wide variety of foods, in all kinds of different colours, is the best way to get a wide variety of nutrients — vitamins, minerals, antioxidants, and all kinds of other essentials we haven't even discovered yet — into your body.

Eating a variety of foods each day will ensure you're getting everything you need for a healthy menstrual cycle. The accompanying chart lists some key nutrients you want to ingest every day and how they affect your health, with a few suggestions on how to get them.

You Can't Out-Supplement a Bad Diet

If you're looking at this list of nutrients and thinking all you have to do to fix your period is pop a few supplements, think again!

Supplements are meant to be just that: *supplemental* to the delicious, nutritious foods that you're eating on a regular basis and that make up most of your diet. Supplements are not silver bullets and they won't let you off the hook when it comes to eating well. You can't out-supplement a crappy diet. I always recommend that you prioritize food over supplements. Fresh, healthy food should be the first source for the nutrients you need in your diet.

Nutrient	How it supports menstrual health	How to get it
Magnesium	Nervous system, blood sugar balance, inflammation, relaxes muscles for cramps and headaches, PMS	Green leafy vegetables, pumpkin seeds, dark chocolate, spinach, swiss chard, sesame seeds, black beans, quinoa
B-complex	Nervous system, regulates stress response, PMS, heavy periods, perimenopause, hormonal balance, mental health	Tuna, turkey, beef, lamb, chicken, salmon, sweet potato, potatoes, sunflower seeds, spinach, bananas, nutritional yeast, yogurt, eggs
Vitamin D	Hormonal health, bone health, blood sugar regulation, immune response	Sunshine, salmon, eggs, mushrooms
Iodine	Supports thyroid, PMS, breast pain, fibroids, heavy periods, cysts, perimenopause	Iodized salt, wild sea food, kelp and seaweed, yogurt, eggs
Zinc	PMS, promotes ovulation, PCOS, endometriosis, painful periods	Pumpkin seeds, sesame seeds, oysters, spinach, mushrooms, beef
Selenium	PMS, endometriosis, cysts, thyroid	Brazil nuts, salmon, mushrooms, asparagus, eggs, barley
Probiotics	Supports gut health and digestion, PMS, endometriosis, estrogen dominance	Fermented foods — miso, kombucha, sauerkraut, kimchi, yogurt, lacto-fermented pickles, kefir, tempeh
Omega essential fatty acids	Inflammation, pain	Hemp seeds, chia seeds, flax, fish oil, evening primrose

However, if you are experiencing specific symptoms that are linked to a deficiency of a vitamin, mineral, or other essential nutrient, then you may require a therapeutic dose — that is, more than what you'll get from food alone — to get your levels back to where they need to be. And if you are a vegan or vegetarian, they are definitely essential.

There are some specific nutrients that can help to balance your hormones and improve your menstrual experience. PMS, for example, has been linked with several nutrient deficiencies, so there is good evidence that nutrition can improve our menstrual experience.

A naturopath, nutritionist, or functional medicine specialist can help you determine what the best supplements are for you, based on your symptoms and lab results.

When buying supplements, purchase the highest quality that you can afford, preferably from a health food store or reputable online dispensary.

SEED CYCLING

The seed cycling protocol is one of my favourite ways to improve your period experience. While it seems too easy to be true, I promise you it really works. I have used it personally and have recommended it to countless clients, family members, and friends seeking period support — and it works every time.

Seed cycling is a naturopathic protocol that involves simply adding a combination of seeds to your diet during each phase of your menstrual cycle — flax and pumpkin during your follicular phase; sesame and sunflower in the luteal phase. It can help with a number of period-related concerns, including irregular cycles, amenorrhea (or absent cycles), PMS, and heavy bleeding.

While there have been no double-blind control studies that prove or disprove the effectiveness of seed cycling for hormone-related issues, the reason why it works makes sense. The nutrients in the seeds support hormonal health. There is also some suggestion that simply bringing mindful attention to your menstrual cycle can help improve its regularity. From my perspective, if something works, do we need to know why? Plus, adding a few tablespoons of seeds to your daily diet certainly isn't going to be harmful.

The one caveat when it comes to seed cycling is that in the same way you can't out-supplement a poor diet, you can't seed cycle it away either. Throwing a couple of tablespoons of ground seeds onto a plate of french fries isn't going to transform your hormonal health. You'll find much greater benefits from getting rid of the junk food and focusing on eating more plants and whole foods than you will the sprinkling of seeds.

TIPS FOR SEED CYCLING

There's no need to make any huge changes to your diet to add in seed cycling: simply add them to whatever you're already eating. Throw them in your smoothie, top a salad or bowl of soup with them — you can even just eat them straight if that's your thing. What's important to remember is that the seeds should be raw and unheated so as not to destroy the delicate nutrients and oils contained in the seeds.

Buy your seeds in small amounts from a well-stocked bulk section that rotates their selection on a regular basis to ensure freshness. Keep them in the fridge or freezer, and if you're grinding them, grind only what you're going to use in the next day or so to maintain the freshness and nutritional integrity of your seeds.

Follicular Phase — Day 1 to Ovulation/New Moon to the Full Moon

During the first half of your cycle until the day that you ovulate (approximately day one to fourteen for those with a twenty-eight-day cycle), or on the new moon, consume one tablespoon of raw flax seeds and one tablespoon of raw pumpkin seeds every day.

Both flax and pumpkin seeds are a source of omega-3 essential fatty acids. Our body needs EFAs to manufacture hormones. Flax seeds also contain lignans, a phytoestrogen, that can help to block excess estrogen in the body. Pumpkin seeds are high in zinc, which is essential for progesterone production.

Luteal Phase — Ovulation to the First Day of Your Next Period/Full Moon to New Moon

During the second phase of your cycle (approximately day fourteen to day twenty-eight for those with a twenty-eight-day cycle) or on the full moon, switch to consuming one tablespoon of raw sesame seeds and one tablespoon of raw sunflower seeds every day.

Sesame and sunflower seeds are high in omega-6 essential fatty acids; these balance out the omega 3 essential fatty acids that we consumed in the first half of the cycle, and are needed to manufacture hormones.

> ### USING SEED CYCLING FOR IRREGULAR CYCLES
>
> If you have an irregular cycle or a very long cycle, then you can align your seed cycling to the phases of the moon rather than menstrual cycle phases. Women have long believed that their menstrual cycles are in sync with the moon — the moon cycle is twenty-eight days long. If you are looking to regulate or shorten your menstrual cycles, the new moon would be considered day one. Note that this has less to do with your menstrual cycle having anything to do with the moon and more to do with bringing a regular rhythm to your cycles.

Like flax seeds, sesame seeds are high in lignans and again will block excess estrogen which can contribute to period issues. Sesame seeds are also high in vitamin E, an essential vitamin for fertility.

Sunflower seeds contain selenium, an essential mineral needed to support our livers, which is a critical organ in producing sex hormones.

Seeds are also a great source of fibre, needed to support digestion and gut health.

HOW YOUR CYCLE AFFECTS YOUR APPETITE

Remember that hormones have an effect on much more than just your menstrual cycle or sex drive — they are also responsible for regulating appetite, among many, many other things. Where you are in your cycle can influence the kinds of foods that you are craving and your ability to choose healthier foods over less fatty foods.

In the first half of our cycle, when you are in the follicular phase and estrogen is rising, we have a tendency to choose healthier foods. During the second half of your cycle, in the luteal phase, it's common to crave higher-fat, higher-calorie foods thanks to progesterone. When you think about the role that progesterone plays in our body when it comes to fertility — to nourish and sustain a pregnancy — it makes sense that we would be craving fat and calories during this phase of our cycle. If we were to become pregnant, we would need the extra nutrients to sustain the pregnancy.

However, many of us may feel that we are useless at sticking to a diet during this time. Just a few weeks ago we were eating a healthy diet while we were in the follicular phase, and now it seems that no matter what we do we're craving chips, chocolate, or other high-calorie foods that are often labelled "bad" or "junk food."

As the goal is to move towards body literacy, including when, what, and how much we eat, it's important that we tune in to these cravings and do our best to honour what our body wants. Deprivation is one of the fastest ways to guarantee that we will overindulge, leaving ourselves feeling uncomfortably full and disappointed that we were unable to "control ourselves" to avoid a food that we had labelled bad. Learning how to eat with an intuitive approach can help us avoid these situations and instead eat the foods we crave in a way that is healthy and sustainable.

Eating a handful of chocolate-covered almonds when you're PMSing isn't going to undo all the hard work you've put in to balance your hormonal health. And don't forget the role that pleasure and joy play in balancing our hormones!

Ensuring that we are well nourished — getting enough calories and taking in a wide variety of nutrients every day of our cycles — can make those PMS cravings easier to deal with. Food cravings may be linked to nutrient deficiencies.

Keeping blood sugar balanced throughout your cycle can also help to buffer cravings, especially cravings for sugar or simple, refined carbohydrates. When your blood sugar is balanced and not riding the wave of spikes and crashes, you are less likely to have intense cravings for sugar or carbohydrates, as your body isn't looking for the quickest source of energy it can find to keep you standing.

When you're in the second half of your cycle, there's no reason why you shouldn't "indulge" in the foods that you're craving. After all, there's room for all foods in a healthy diet.

WHEN GREEN JUICE ISN'T ENOUGH

As a nutritionist, I believe in the power of food. I know first hand, from my own personal experience and the experiences of my clients, that what we eat — and how — can make a big difference when it comes to our health and our day-to-day wellness. At the same time, I'm also realistic, and I recognize that food is only one part of a very large and very complex equation.

Here's some real talk: there are going to be scenarios when food — even when it's the healthiest, most nutrient-dense food on the planet — isn't going to be enough.

If you suffer from a disease like endometriosis or your infertility challenges are the result of a blocked uterine tube, no amount of green juice is going to cure it, reverse it, or take it away. Your food choices might help you manage your symptoms, but at the end of the day you'll still have endo or whatever disease you might be suffering from.

Jessica Murnane, founder of Know Your Endo, said it best: "When you have endo, no amount of green juice is going to stop that bitch from coming back."[7]

So, while I believe that there is always value in taking a nutritional approach to our health and wellness, I am also realistic about how far it can take us.

CHAPTER 9
STRESS AND YOUR MENSTRUAL CYCLE

I'm going to say this in no uncertain terms: stress messes with your hormones and your menstrual cycles.

As you start to tune in to your body, you may notice that as your hormones fluctuate throughout your menstrual cycle, so do your energy levels and mood. The grind of modern society doesn't account for the literal and figurative ebbs and flows of the body, and especially the menstrual cycle; we are expected to feel the same each and every day. Our society values productivity over the cyclic nature of the seasons and our bodies.

These days, the nine to five is more like the eight to six, or maybe even seven or eight at night, plus answering emails well into the evening. Add on the demands of parenting, caring for aging parents, and the emotional labour at home and in the workplace that so often falls into the laps of modern women and femme-presenting people — deep stuff like lending a shoulder to cry on, and the superficial stuff, too, like celebrating office birthdays, making a grocery list, and remembering who needs to be picked up where and at what time. Top all that with a relentless, twenty-four-hour, seven-days-a-week cycle of seemingly endless bad news and constant notifications from our smartphones and it's no wonder we're left stressed out and chronically overstimulated. We're relying on adrenaline and cortisol, hormones that are supposed to be for acute, short-term stress, to get us through these long days. Then, when we finally get to bed at night, we're exhausted but totally wired and unable to fall asleep.

As a wellness practitioner, I'm well aware of how stress affects our health — menstrual or otherwise. It's a key factor in just about every major disease progression from heart disease to cancer.

However, as an entrepreneur and parent, I also know that being told to "manage my stress" is BS. Not to mention offensive. And it's also the fastest way to get me to walk out of your office and never come back.

Telling women that they need to slow down is just another instrument of the patriarchy — it's a micro-aggression that harkens back to outdated ideas of femininity and gender roles. Do what you want and what you need to! But achievements, whether they be in your career, academics, sport, or your personal life, shouldn't come at the expense of your health. Body literacy is an act of resistance, and self-care is, too — not in the manicures and bubble-bath kind of way, but in the asserting personal boundaries way. In fact, tuning into your body and its natural rhythms can actually help you do more while also getting the rest and relaxation that you need. I'll explore this in the following chapters.

The fact is, stress and chronic overstimulation, which is the result of never being able to turn off that stress or reset our nervous system, makes us sick — mentally, physically, perhaps even spiritually. It's not working hard, doing the work, going after our dreams, balancing a family (or not) with a career (or not), or paying our dues that makes stress so toxic. It's never giving our bodies a chance to come down from the adrenaline rush and reset that makes stress so harmful.

So, let me be clear about this, too. It's not that you need to do less. Instead, you need to find a way to buffer that stress and lower your load. Just like the endocrine-disrupting chemicals and other toxins that overload your liver, you'll never be completely free of them until someone invents a way to breathe organic air. And unless you're planning to move away to an ashram in India, you're likely never going to be completely stress-free, either. Instead, you need to build resilience to stress by turning the stress response off, and resetting.

WHAT IS STRESS?

Our bodies experience two kinds of stress. There's external stress, the stuff you might typically associate with stress like work deadlines, family obligations, rent cheques, and the news cycle. Your body also experiences stress from the blue light of your phone screen or TV, from Wi-Fi signals, from the sound of a fire truck screaming outside of your window... anything that kicks your nervous system into high alert.

On top of all that, there's internal stress — stress that comes from inside your body, often by eating pro-inflammatory foods, foods that are irritating to our guts, things that are difficult to digest or simply don't agree with our constitution because we are sensitive or allergic to them.

Exposure to endocrine disrupting chemicals and carcinogens in the environment and in our homes from plastic and cleaning and personal care products like makeup, shampoo, and hand sanitizer also puts stress on your body. What you put on your skin doesn't just stay there; it's absorbed through your skin and into your bloodstream. Your body then mounts an inflammatory immune response to deal with the toxic load, which also kicks your stress response into gear.

It's an assault from all sides. An appropriate analogy would be a cartoon character sticking their finger in a light socket; their hair is standing up on end while electricity pulses through their body. They are literally fried. With all of the stimulation of the modern world from both internal and external stressors, we are, too.

HOW DOES YOUR BODY RESPOND TO STRESS?

When your body senses that you might be in some sort of danger (i.e., stress), your nervous system kicks in to do what it needs to in order to protect you and keep you alive. We have two parts to our nervous system: the parasympathetic and the sympathetic.

The sympathetic nervous system is responsible for the "fight-or-flight" response to stress. It causes your muscles to contract and your heart rate to increase. Hormones are pumped into your bloodstream so that you can either fight for your life or run away if you need to. Bodily functions that aren't immediately essential, like reproduction, the immune system, and even digestion, shut down.

Your parasympathetic nervous system increases the production of saliva and digestive enzymes; lowers your heart rate; and relaxes your muscles. After the fight-or-flight response has been activated, the parasympathetic nervous system calms you back down, keeping you humming along and supporting your long-term stress. It restores balance, allowing our bodies to relax and repair — "rest, digest, and make babies" as the saying goes.

But here's the thing about bodies and stress. Your body doesn't know the difference between the stress a human experienced thousands of years ago — like running from a bear — and the stress of a tight work deadline.

(I don't know what you do on the weekends, but I know that I'm much more likely to experience the work deadline than a bear!) From your body's perspective, stress equals imminent danger and a threat to your life. If your body senses that you're not safe, or it's using all of its resources just to keep the lights on, it's going to shut down reproduction — which is the function of the menstrual cycle, after all, even though that's not its only benefit.

Cortisol, one of the most important stress hormones, and progesterone, a key hormone in our menstrual cycles, are both manufactured in the body along the same pathways. The thing is, your body looks at one as optional. And it's not the stress response.

Our stress response isn't something we need to fight against. It's a good thing that we have it; it's kept us safe and out of danger, running from those bears, and has helped us evolve and exist as a species. However, though our bodies are designed to mount a response to stress, they are also supposed to ease up and reset — that's where the parasympathetic nervous system comes in. Ideally, we'd be spending most of our time in this state. However, when we're chronically stressed, that sympathetic nervous system and stress response is always running. Our cortisol levels don't get reset, which means that our adrenal glands are going into overdrive. If we're too busy trying to make enough cortisol to keep up with the demands of chronic stress, there won't be an opportunity for the body to produce progesterone, i.e., through ovulation, leading to menstrual disturbances.

STRESS AND YOUR PERIODS

So, maybe it's not news to you that our modern society is stressful and that stress has an enormous impact on your health. More than food or any of the environmental factors that we've discussed so far, chronic stress can wreak the most havoc on your cycle. After all, your menstrual cycle is a vital sign, too.

Your hypothalamus gland, located in your brain, is incredibly sensitive to stress and environmental factors. It is the gland responsible for telling your pituitary gland to release follicle-stimulating hormone and luteinizing hormone, the two hormones that trigger ovulation. If your hypothalamus senses that you're stressed out, this will put the brakes on ovulation. If you're not ovulating, you're not going to get your period. The result could be long, irregular cycles, or even absent periods.

If you've ever noticed that your period was late after a stressful time — even if it was good stress, like travelling abroad or starting your dream job — this is why. Your body may have cycled right up to the moments before ovulation, but it didn't cross the finish line because of stress: your hypothalamus prohibited the release of the hormones needed to allow the egg to be released. If the pressure eased off, you might ovulate a few days later when your body tries again. Your follicular phase will be extended, causing your period to show up a few days later than expected.

I recently met a woman who was concerned that her periods had recently disappeared. The first question I asked was about what was going on in her life over the past couple of months. Was it a busy time at work? Right away, she recognized that she had just moved house, which had caused a lot of stress and anxiety. Together we pieced together that the move coincided with when she would normally have ovulated, so it was likely that the stress of the move suppressed her ovulation, which explained why she hadn't gotten her period.

Chronic stress can also contribute to more serious issues with the menstrual cycle. Hypothalamic amenorrhea is a condition that causes your menstrual cycle to stop altogether, meaning you don't ovulate and therefore you don't get a period for at least six months when there is no medical diagnosis, such as PCOS or thyroid disease, to explain the absence.[1]

So how do we get out of the fight-or-flight stress response to support our hormones?

LOWERING THE STRESS LOAD

When I was in nutrition school we talked a lot about "stress management," almost as much as we talked about food, because that's how much stress impacts your health. But in the real world when I started to talk to clients about "managing" their stress, I realized that this wasn't just an abstract concept to them: it was completely bullshit, not to mention insulting. There is nothing that would make me walk out of a practitioner's office faster, and likely never return, then being told to manage my stress by slowing down, taking it easier, or giving up one of my passionate pursuits. As an entrepreneur and parent, I have worked hard for everything I've achieved in my life, and I'm not about to slow down now. This is a quality I also recognize in my clients and those who come to my workshops.

I also recognize the inherent privilege of stress management. A single mother who is working three part-time jobs isn't going to avoid the long-term health effects of stress by "managing" it. Being able to manage the stress in your life often means outsourcing, which is not a choice that is available to everyone.

Lowering your stress load doesn't have to mean hiring a weekly house cleaner. It can be as simple as breathing. Remember the breathing exercises outlined in the "getting to know your body" section of this book? These are useful not just to get to know your body, but to, you know, breathe. A couple of deep breaths doesn't cost a cent, and it's not going to add any more time to your day. It might seem too simple, but I promise it will have a profound effect on resetting your nervous system and lifting your mood. Chances are you're probably unconsciously taking a few deep breaths right now as you read these words. And if you're not, give it a try. I'll wait....

So, when it comes to stress, it might not be about slowing down, giving things up, or passing up opportunities — it's about cutting out the crap that we can do without (when we can) and making time to get out of fight-or-flight mode to intentionally unwind and reset your stress response. Not only will that help to chill us out — it leaves room for creativity and passion to spark future projects and endeavours.

As we'll see in the final section of this book, this creative energy may be tied to your ovulation and menstrual cycles. So, there's another bonus reason to support your hormonal health and make sure that you're ovulating on a regular basis. You want to be able to tap into that place of creativity and creative energy!

For better or for worse, living in the modern world comes with a certain amount of stress baked into it. You're always going to have deadlines at work, family obligations, daycare bills, the commute to and from work; but is there anything in your life that is optional that might be causing your stress level to skyrocket? Often women take on more than they need to out of obligation — we often take on responsibilities that we don't want because we've been conditioned not to want to disappoint others.

The first step in lowering the stress in our lives is to take a good, hard look at where that stress is coming from. Is it actually the Sunday night family dinners you're obligated to attend every week? Or is it the volunteer work that you begrudgingly took on, even though you didn't want to, and which you inevitably leave until after your Sunday night family dinner to finish that is stressing you out? Maybe feeling stressed out about that obligation makes you resentful of the other obligations that, in reality, you actually enjoy.

Getting clear on your priorities and values can help bring these types of tensions into focus. What is it that you value in this season of life? Is it volunteer work or family time? If the answer is both, then you need to find a way to create and uphold a boundary that allows you to do both.

We might not all be able to quit our day jobs — and I'd never suggest that as the cure-all for everybody — but chances are, there are things in your life that are causing you stress that you could get rid of, whether it's obligations that no longer serve you, a toxic relationship, an energy vampire who leaves you feeling drained and tired, or a bad habit. These are the types of stressful things that we often *do* have control over. So, get rid of what you can control and see what that does for your stress level.

Then learn to create boundaries around the sources of stress that you can't cut out of your life. I'm passionate about the work that I do, but I find myself getting resentful about my work when I'm scrolling through emails on my phone while simultaneously trying to get dinner fixed and wrangle a tired, hungry toddler who's just come home from a long day at preschool. For a long time, I assumed that the only way out of this was to work less, get more childcare, or hire a meal service — or better yet, all three. But when I really sat down to think about it, I realized that the answer was to not scroll through emails on my phone while simultaneously trying to get dinner fixed and wrangle a tired, hungry toddler.

It wasn't the work and it wasn't the home and family obligations that was causing tension. Allowing my boundaries to be porous, meaning that I allowed work time and family time to overlap in a way that wasn't actually productive or making me feel good, is where that stress came from. Putting down my phone for half an hour while I make dinner and spend time with my kid didn't cost me any money.

While lowering your stress load and creating boundaries isn't going to necessarily lighten your heavy flow or relieve your menstrual cramps immediately, it will have a long-term effect on your hormonal health when your stress response is lower and your hormones are in balance. Committing to improving your hormonal health and your periods is a long game and not one that is going to be won with quick fixes.

REST, DIGEST, AND PRACTISE SELF-CARE

When I say practise self-care, what I mean is *do something to intentionally unwind and de-stress* — switch off the sympathetic nervous system and get into the parasympathetic rest and digest mode.

One of my nutrition school teachers actually called the parasympathetic nervous system "rest and digest and make babies" in order to highlight the importance this body system has on ovulation and fertility. In the old days, this was called leisure or relaxation. While stress has a detrimental effect on so many facets of our health and wellness, being able to reset from that stress is crucial for mitigating its negative effects.

Social media has co-opted self-care into just another thing that we are expected to do picture-perfectly, which in turn contributes to our stress levels and overstimulation! Never mind what's going to look good on Instagram. What's going to bring you a little joy and make you feel amazing?

Self-care is more than just bubble baths. It's asserting the boundaries we discussed earlier. It's taking care of your physical, mental, and emotional self. It's self-preservation, as Audre Lorde said.

Taking care of yourself isn't just an act of self-care, no matter how it's defined, but more like self-parenting. You tell a child to get to bed on time because they need to be well rested for school, to eat their vegetables because the nutrients are good for them. We really need to start taking our own advice and talking to ourselves more like children in an effort to self-parent. You don't want to go to bed? You don't want to eat your vegetables? Ask yourself how you'd speak to a child who was protesting in the same way and follow through accordingly.

FINDING PLEASURE AND JOY

Another way to avoid the self-care-as-to-do-list-item trap is to reframe it as seeking pleasure and joy. Give yourself permission to do things just because you like them and they make you happy. It's easy to get caught up in what we *have* to do — we *have to* get to work on time, we *have to* be a certain way or act in a particular way. What we *want* to do can sometimes get obscured.

We all have our own ways to bring joy and pleasure into our lives; this can have a profound effect on our hormonal health — it helps us to relax, boosts self-esteem, and increases feelings of well-being all around.

TWENTY IDEAS FOR PLEASURE AND SELF-CARE
THAT DON'T INVOLVE A BUBBLE BATH

We're all grown-ups here, and maybe we don't need a checklist for how to have fun or create pleasure in our lives. But then again, maybe we do. Modern lives are busy and stressful, and if we're caught in a chronic stress loop trying to come up with something to do for FUN and JOY, that may actually give us more anxiety. Hence why I keep my Pleasure List. So here I present twenty different ideas for creating pleasure and joy while cultivating self-care in your life — no bubble baths included:

1. Taking a few deep breaths
2. Saying no
3. Going for a walk
4. Meditating
5. Listening to your favourite music (and singing out loud)
6. Dancing
7. Having an orgasm — on your own or with a partner!
8. Lighting a candle or diffusing your favourite scent
9. Turning off your phone
10. Taking a break
11. Unfollowing anyone who makes you feel like crap on social media
12. Buying yourself flowers
13. Tidying up your workspace
14. Making a home-cooked meal (or ordering takeout)
15. Calling friends or family to catch up
16. Going to bed early
17. Drinking water
18. Wearing whatever makes you feel best
19. Reading
20. Practising your hobby, craft, or sport

The more time we spend in "rest and digest" mode, the healthier we will be, hormones included.

Think about what brings you pleasure. I'm not just talking about sex; it could be anything that makes *you* feel good. For me, a smear of lipstick brings me pleasure. So does diffusing essential oils in my office while I write. I keep a page in my journal called "The Pleasure List" that I add to on a regular basis whenever I feel that super juicy, good feeling of joy. Dancing, family walks to nowhere in particular, a long shower, wearing matching underwear, and clean sheets are all on that list. When I'm not feeling at my best, it's a good way to get some inspiration for how to shift my mood.

What you do to unwind is far less important than the fact that you are simply making time to relax and blow off steam — provided that what you are doing is legal and safe, of course.

LOWER YOUR INTERNAL STRESS LOAD

Stress doesn't just come from the outside; it also comes from within — largely because of what we eat and our gut health. Eating pro-inflammatory foods or foods that we are sensitive to, or not adequately chewing our food, can all promote inflammation in our gut lining, which in turn can lead to adverse symptoms that show up in our menstrual cycles and elsewhere. Riding the constant rise and fall of sugar highs and crashes can also contribute to internal stress. We can lower our internal stress load by being mindful of blood sugar regulation, chewing our food, and eliminating inflammatory foods. Identifying which foods we may be sensitive or allergic to can also help lower this load.

BE MINDFUL OF OVERSTIMULATION

A key signal for me that I am stressed out is that I'm reaching for my phone first thing in the morning and I'm staring at a screen, zombie-like, until well past my bedtime.

However, blue light from computer screens, phones, and TVs interrupts our sleep by messing with the production and release of a key sleep hormone known as melatonin. So many of us are now in front of screens all day, which keeps you stimulated well into the night when you want to be asleep. At the end of a long day, instead of scrolling through Instagram as you're trying to drift off to sleep, shut down your TV, phone, and computer at least an hour before bedtime.

Use this time to read, get ready for bed, listen to a guided meditation, have an orgasm by yourself or with a partner — or my personal favourite, just lie in bed and stare at the ceiling!

If you do use a screen in the evenings, use night-time mode or an app like f.lux that replaces the hormone-disrupting blue light of the screen with a yellow hue that's easier on your eyes and doesn't mess with your hormones.

MANAGING THE STRESS OF MAKING POSITIVE CHANGES

If you have been suffering from period-related pain or other menstrual symptoms for some time, the idea that there is relief in sight can be exciting: you want to start right away making changes to your diet, exercise routine, stress management — and you're learning to chart. Jumping in with two feet can be overwhelming, creating *more* stress in your life; the last thing you want to do when it comes to hormonal health.

I know this from personal experience. When I transitioned off birth control, I was doing all the things. I was excited to finally be having a natural cycle and one that wasn't leaving me with debilitating headaches. I was learning to chart and tracking as many signs of fertility as I could; taking my temperature each morning; making changes to what I was eating; exercising; wearing a fitness tracker; meditating; and journaling. Although I was starting to feel better than I ever had before, I was also starting to feel burnt out. All of my free time was spent on managing my health. While I might have been feeling better, I was boring even myself.

One thing that was particularly stressing me out was the fact that my temperatures were never showing up where they "should" be on my charts. Low body temperatures can be linked to low thyroid function. I was aware of this and starting each day frustrated. Not getting my temperatures "right" was taking a toll. When my naturopathic doctor suggested that I pull back on doing *all* the things, and in particular taking my temperatures, it felt like a huge weight had been lifted off my shoulders.

So, when it comes to making changes, do what feels right to you; do what feels manageable. Sometimes big, sweeping changes can do more harm than good. Picking one or two easy changes that are sustainable will have a big impact over time. Whatever you're doing, keeping a journal to track your day-to-day progress can help you to see the bigger picture a little more clearly. It's easy to get impatient when it comes to hormonal health improvements given that it's a marathon, not a sprint. It's going to take time before you see changes. This can be frustrating, particularly if you're making changes to support fertility. But keep your eye on the prize!

CHAPTER 10

OTHER LIFESTYLE FACTORS FOR BETTER PERIODS

Taking a holistic approach to health and healing — regardless of whether you're looking to support your hormones and periods, or any other health issue — means more than just looking at the foods that you eat. Other lifestyle factors, like exercise, sleep, and, when it comes to your period, the types of menstrual products that you use, also contribute to your hormonal health.

EXERCISE

Just as the news that eating vegetables is good for you wasn't exactly, well, *news*, I am sure that the same is true when I tell you that exercise comes with a multitude of health benefits when it comes to your period. These benefits include lowering cortisol and regulating your stress response, increasing blood flow to your pelvis, and reducing chronic inflammation. It's also been shown to have a positive effect on reducing the physical symptoms of PMS and dysmenorrhea. Just twenty minutes of aerobic exercise three times a week can reduce PMS symptoms.[1]

It can be difficult to get moving when you're not feeling your best or when you're in pain. I get that. In the same way that nutrition supports your menstrual experience all days of your cycle, the same goes for exercise. Exercise at any point in your cycle will likely have a positive effect on your symptoms. And if you're in the habit of exercising the other weeks of your cycle, it will be that much easier to get moving.

You can use an intuitive approach to choose your exercise or movement practice, just like you can with eating. What do you *like* to do? What is your body telling you that it needs right now in terms of exercise and movement? Tune in, listen to what your body needs, and then do that. There's no single way to exercise that's right for everyone, and what you need in terms of exercise can change from day to day and week to week in your cycle. When you're menstruating, you might find that your energy is lower, and a brisk walk and some light stretching is just what you need. Other times when your energy is higher, a more intense workout like yoga flow or spinning is challenging and satisfying in all the right ways.

Like anything, it is possible to have too much of a good thing. This is especially true when it comes to menstrual and hormonal health and exercise. Extreme over-exercising can even stop your periods altogether. Amenorrhea together with eating disorders and low bone mineral density are known as the *female athlete triad*, because they are three health issues often found in young female athletes in sports that emphasize leanness or low body weight, such as dance, figure skating, or gymnastics.

But you don't need to be training for the Olympics for exercise to have an adverse effect on your periods. Intense exercise, particularly with a high cardio component, kicks in your body's stress response. It then produces cortisol, which will have a downstream effect on your menstrual cycle and may lead to delayed ovulation, irregular periods, or even absent periods.

However, that's not a get-out-of-gym-class-free card. If you're doing high-intensity workouts five or six days a week and you're noticing changes or irregularities with your menstrual cycle, it might be time to pull that back a little.

In the previous chapter I recommended building de-stress techniques into your lifestyle, rather than lessening your ambitions. It's the same thing here. If you love intense workouts you don't have to give them up, just make time to buffer those high-intensity workouts with lower-impact exercise that will help to reset and regulate your stress response. So, swap out one of your weekly CrossFit sessions for a yoga or Pilates class, a hike, or even just some simple stretching. You'll still get all of the benefits of exercise without compromising your hormonal health.

ENDOCRINE-DISRUPTING CHEMICALS

Endocrine-disrupting chemicals (EDC) are found in our environment, as well as in cleaning products, personal care products, pesticides, and other household concoctions, and they have an effect on our hormonal health.

The name says it all — they disrupt our endocrine system. This can happen in many different ways, such as increasing or decreasing production of certain hormones; imitating or interfering with hormone signalling; turning one hormone into another; or even competing with essential nutrients.

The Environmental Working Group, a non-profit, non-partisan organization dedicated to protecting human health and the environment, identified the twelve endocrine-disrupting chemicals that are most prevalent:

1. BPA
2. Dioxin
3. Atrazine
4. Phthalates
5. Perchlorate
6. Fire retardants
7. Lead
8. Arsenic
9. Mercury
10. Perfluorinated chemicals (PFCs)
11. Organophosphate pesticides
12. Glycol ethers

These chemicals can be found in just about anything — from the BPA and phthalates in plastic, to pesticides like atrazine found in our food and water supply, dioxins in tampons and menstrual products, and fire retardants in furniture and clothing. From the air that we breathe to our homes, chemicals that disrupt our hormonal health can be found just about everywhere.

Toxins and chemicals seem to be divisive, particularly in mainstream media and the medical community. One argument is that the levels of chemicals that you're exposed to in, say, a tampon, is minimal and therefore not of concern. This viewpoint doesn't account for the *toxic load* — you're not going to just use one tampon in your lifetime, you're going to use thousands. And it's not just tampons that are exposing you to chemicals. They're also in the food that you eat, in plastics that are found in just about *everything* these days, and in personal care products and makeup. One study found that the average woman uses a dozen personal care products every day, exposing them to 168 unique chemical ingredients, many of which are known or probable reproductive and developmental toxins linked to infertility.[2] That exposure adds up over time and creates a burden in your body.

Another argument is that even if we *are* exposed to toxic chemicals daily, our bodies have a built-in detox system designed to protect us from the harmful effects. They're right; human bodies absolutely come with a built-in filter and detox system — it's called your liver. Remember that your liver has more than five hundred jobs to do? Well, detoxing is one of them. Hormone production and metabolism is another. If your liver gets overloaded with gunk from the air you're breathing, the food you're eating, and the creams and lotions that you slather on your body, it's going to get congested, and is not going to be functioning at an optimal level. In other words, it's not going to be manufacturing and processing hormones, which may ultimately be reflected in your menstrual cycle.

Reducing our toxic load and the burden on our bodies is essential for our hormonal health.

You might be thinking that if we can't get away from them, perhaps there's no use in trying to avoid them. Like stress, it's not about being 100 percent toxin-free at all times — until they invent a way to produce and breathe organic air, that's simply not going to happen. While the onus shouldn't be on people to navigate which products may contain harmful chemicals and which ones don't, that's currently how it works. I suggest looking for natural and organic cleaning and personal care products and for plastics that are labelled BPA- and phthalates-free (or better yet, switch to glass or stainless steel when possible).

Once again, not everyone has the option to choose these products, either because they're not available or because they often come at a higher price. Progress, not perfection, is the name of the game — some chemical-free products are better than none. And they're not just better for you; they're also better for the environment.

The suggestion isn't that you throw out everything in your makeup drawer or cleaning cupboard and start fresh with brand-new products. But the next time you go to replace your shampoo or mascara, consider purchasing a more natural, chemical-free option. If you're concerned that the natural options don't work as well, I assure you they've come a long way from the patchouli-scented everything you used to find at the health food store. There are numerous options for natural and "clean" beauty, personal care, and cleaning products that rival any chemical-laden, conventional brands out there, and the market is growing — with new brands debuting every day.

And if there's a product that you absolutely, can't possibly ever fathom replacing with something else? That's okay, too; because what you do most of the time matters more than once in a while. That said, you can pry my drugstore hairspray out of my cold, dead hands! I don't recognize a single ingredient on the label, and I'm okay with that. It's not something I use every day, and the rest of my products, from my shampoo to my makeup, and even my household cleaning products, are clean and green.

CHOOSING BETTER MENSTRUAL PRODUCTS, FOR YOU AND THE ENVIRONMENT

For better or for worse, menstrual management products are a fact of life — they do play an important role in health and hygiene. Unfortunately, the products that many of us use expose us to harmful chemicals, create an incredible amount of waste that is damaging our environment, and may be contributing to our period pains, UTIs, yeast infections, and other pelvic-related disorders.

Menstrual product manufacturers aren't currently required to disclose the ingredients in their products, so it's hard to know what you're putting in or next to one of the most sensitive parts of your body. While consumer pressure in recent years has led to some manufacturers voluntarily disclosing what's in their products, that likely doesn't include information about any of the ingredients or chemicals that were used in their processing and packaging.

Many conventional menstrual management products, such as pads and tampons, are processed with bleach, fragrance, and other harsh chemicals that you probably don't want in or near your vagina.

A study conducted by Women's Voices for the Earth in 2018 tested six popular tampon brands for chemicals; four were conventional brands and two were natural, organic brands. Of the conventional brands, all four were found to include at least one known carcinogenic ingredient. Among them was carbon disulphide, which is commonly used in the production of rayon. Exposure to carbon disulphide has been associated with an increased risk of menstrual disorders, early menopause, and hormone disturbances.[3]

Think about it for a second. When you're putting potentially toxic chemicals into an area that is already incredibly sensitive and prone to inflammation, it's only going to increase that inflammation, which in turn may increase pain and discomfort. It's like rubbing salt into the wound.

Once again, those who oppose the use of natural, organic, or reusable products claim that the exposure to chemicals in a tampon or pad is slight. But this assertion doesn't take into account the number of products that you'll use over the course of your entire menstruating life, or the other ways in which you're exposed to chemicals in your everyday life. It all adds up. Plus, there is no research on the potential health impacts from vaginal exposure to chemicals often found in menstrual management products, so it's impossible to say how much exposure is safe.

If you are suffering from painful periods, switching to a non-toxic product like a menstrual cup or natural, all-cotton tampons or pads is worth a try. It may reduce your inflammation and in turn any pain you may be experiencing, and at the very least, will be healthier for you and the environment.

Something that I hear time and time again from friends, clients, podcast guests, and in forums on the internet is that making the switch from conventional tampons to natural brands or a reusable product such as a menstrual cup can drastically reduce pain and cramping. Personally, the cramps I had been experiencing when using tampons virtually disappeared after making the switch to a cup.

When it comes to period products, we don't just have the health and safety of our own health to consider, but that of the planet, too. Given the environmental crisis our world is in today, we no longer have the luxury of ignoring the waste associated with menstrual management products: many of these products are made from and packaged in plastic. And we're only talking about the products themselves — who knows what kinds of materials and chemicals go into the manufacturing, packaging, and shipping process. A small package of conventional pads contains as much plastic as three plastic shopping bags! That's a lot of plastic that's not making it into the recycling bin, I'm sure.

On average you'll use thousands of tampons or pads over the course of your menstruating life — as in eleven thousand-ish, perhaps more if you have a long or heavy flow — and just because they've been flushed or thrown away doesn't mean that they've disappeared; they've just been relocated to landfills or waterways where they'll eventually wash up on beaches. I've heard some people jokingly refer to tampon applicators as "beach whistles."

Menstrual products should be safe — for the person using it and for the environment. If you have the choice, then it seems like a clear one: choose organic, natural, or better yet, reusable products for managing your period blood. And make sure your voice is heard as to why you've made the switch. Let the companies that are making and distributing these products know that you won't purchase products that may be harmful by calling them out on social media, writing a letter or email, or phoning their customer support line. Don't let them think that your dollars don't matter. They do!

Luckily, today we have more choice when it comes to menstrual management products than ever before. Natural and organic options for pads and tampons are more accessible in health food stores and many mainstream drugstores and are more affordable than they have been in the past. Not to mention the wide variety of subscription services that will deliver a customized box of products directly to your door, once a month, perfectly timed with the arrival of your period. Reusable products, once reserved for only the most crunchy-granola hippies, have gone mainstream in recent years thanks to savvy marketing that appeals to millennial shoppers looking for hip products that will also be better for the environment and their own health. Menstrual cups, reusable pads, and period underwear — underwear that has a reusable, absorbent pad built right in — are all better options for both you and the environment.

Your wallet will thank you too. While there is an upfront cost to reusable menstrual products, they can last for several years, saving you money in the long run. A menstrual cup priced around $30 pays for itself in just a couple of months.

Here's a breakdown of menstrual management products and a guide for choosing the one that's best for you.

Disposable Pads

Probably the most accessible in terms of use and availability, disposable pads come in a variety of sizes, shapes, and absorbencies, in conventional brands and natural and organic brands. Disposable pads adhere to the gusset of your underwear with a sticky adhesive, with or without "wings" that wrap around to hold it in place. Depending on the absorbency level and your flow, they can be worn between four to eight hours. If possible, I recommend choosing natural and/or organic brands that use as little plastic packaging as possible.

Cloth Pads

As exposure to chemicals and the environment become more of a concern, cloth pads have been enjoying a resurgence. They work in just the same way as a disposable pad but are made of soft fabrics like cotton, hemp, or bamboo, and can be washed and dried after each use and worn again. There are a wide variety of manufacturers selling cloth pads online in all the shapes and sizes that you would expect from a disposable pad, from a thong-friendly liner to an overnight or postpartum pad. Each brand works a little differently — some have absorbable liners sewn directly into the pad while others use a pocket system that allows you to insert liners and change the absorbency as needed. Depending on your flow and what's comfortable for you, a cloth pad can be worn just like a disposable — about four to six hours. When you're done, rinse in cold water and follow the manufacturer's instructions for washing and drying.

If you're crafty, you can find plenty of patterns for sewing your own cloth pads at home, a great way to upcycle old clothes or materials that you're no longer using.

Interlabial Pads

These small petal- or leaf-shaped reusable pads are made of soft, absorbent material like terry cloth or flannel. Worn outside of the vagina, they are held in place by the outer labia and are an alternative to both pads and tampons as a sort of in-between. While generally not available commercially, there are lots of makers on websites like Etsy that are selling interlabial pads. File these pads under the "alternative" category, although I was surprised to learn that many *Heavy Flow* listeners swear by them; particularly those who tend to "gush" — if you know what I mean. Interlabial pads should be changed every four to six hours, rinsed in cold water, and washed and dried according to the manufacturer's directions.

Tampons

Worn internally, tampons are made of cotton, rayon, or a blend and absorb menstrual blood in the vagina. There are many brands available in a variety of absorbencies, with or without applicators, in both conventional and natural/organic brands. Absorbency levels are regulated across all brands. For example, a super plus tampon will absorb between twelve millilitres and sixteen millilitres no matter what brand you choose. That goes for both conventional drugstore brands and natural or organic ones.

If you choose to use tampons, always choose the lowest absorbency needed for your flow and change them often (every four to six hours) to reduce the risk of toxic shock syndrome. For example, if you have a light flow, use a light absorbency tampon. It's always better to err on the side of caution and use a lower absorbency one changed more often or with a back-up pad or liner.

Menstrual Cups

These small cups are made of medical-grade materials such as silicone and are designed to be worn in the vaginal canal, collecting rather than absorbing menstrual blood. They can be worn for up to twelve hours, then rinsed and reused. Empty the contents of your cup into the toilet and wash your hands and the cup with a mild soap before reinserting. Cups can also be wiped up with toilet paper in a pinch. At the end of your cycle, pop your cup into boiling water for five to ten minutes to sterilize it before the next use. With proper care they can be used for several years. When it's time to dispose of a silicone menstrual cup, it can be burned down to ash.

Having gained popularity in recent years as people become more aware of the health and environmental concerns related to conventional pads and tampons, there are now many different cups on the market. Many people mistakenly think that "cups aren't for them" after trying a single cup, not knowing that there are different shapes and sizes that might work better for them. I recommend visiting putacupinit.com and taking their quiz to find the perfect cup for you.

Although cups collect rather than absorb menstrual blood, they still carry a risk of toxic shock syndrome (TSS). A 2018 study confirmed that bacteria that cause TSS can grow on a menstrual cup,[4] and there has been one reported death from TSS linked to a menstrual cup.[5] To reduce the risk of TSS when using a menstrual cup, make sure to change it frequently, washing both the cup and your hands with soap and water, and boil in between uses. You can also have two cups in rotation to further reduce the risk. And always take care when inserting or removing the cup to avoid breaking the skin inside of the vagina, which increases the risk of bacteria entering your body.

Menstrual Discs

Similar to a menstrual cup in that it collects rather than absorbs menstrual blood, discs are worn just under the cervix and are held in place with the pubic bone — this space is called the fornix and is the widest part of the vagina — rather than in the vaginal canal where a menstrual cup sits. Menstrual discs come in both reusable and disposable styles and can be worn for several hours. One of the selling points for menstrual discs is that they can be worn for mess-free penetrative period sex because they keep the vaginal canal clear.

Period Underwear

Imagine a pair of underwear that has absorbent material built right in so you don't need to use an additional product to manage your menstrual flow. That's exactly what period underwear is. It's been gaining popularity in recent years, particularly since 2015 when New York City–based period underwear brand Thinx made headlines with their period-positive subway ads. Like cloth pads, each brand and style is a little different, with absorbent layers sewn in or with a pocket system where you insert liners for more or less absorbency. Just about every style of underwear is now available with period protection, from hipster shorts to thongs and gender-neutral boxers or briefs, making them an excellent choice for the trans or non-binary menstruator. Some brands have even started making period-proof bathing suits for hitting the beach or pool!

Depending on your flow and the absorbency of the underwear, it can be worn for several hours. After use, rinse in cold water and wash and dry according to the manufacturer's directions.

Sea Sponges

Natural sponges from the sea can be inserted into the vagina to absorb menstrual blood. They can be worn for about six to eight hours and reused for three to six cycles or months. After you remove it, rinse it out to wash away the blood before reinserting. At the end of your cycle the sponge needs to be washed thoroughly to sanitize it. The benefits of sea sponges are that they are sustainable and biodegradable. Sea sponges can also be worn during penetrative intercourse for mess-free period sex.

Note that the FDA hasn't approved sea sponges for use as a menstrual management product. Sponges are live organisms that come from the sea and may contain bacteria, sand, and other nasty things — including the bacteria that causes toxic shock syndrome — although many menstruators looking for an all-natural product swear by them! If you try them out, look for an established retailer that specifically markets their sponges for menstrual management, change them regularly, and follow care instructions carefully.

REDUCING THE RISK OF TOXIC SHOCK SYNDROME

If you choose a menstrual product that is worn internally, it's important to be aware of the risks of toxic shock syndrome (TSS), even if you're using natural or organic tampons or a menstrual cup. TSS is caused by the bacterial toxins Streptococcus pyogenes or Staphylococcus aureus. When these toxins get into the bloodstream, they can cause illness, generally described as flu-like symptoms, which can be deadly.

Tampons absorb all of the moisture in the vaginal canal, not just menstrual blood. This can potentially dry out the skin in the vagina, which can cause microtears in the skin and leave you susceptible to infection. Bacteria can enter the bloodstream through these microtears and make you sick. Make sure that you choose the lowest absorbency for your flow (using a higher absorbency can dry out the vagina) and change your tampon frequently.

While menstrual cups collect rather than absorb menstrual flow, there is still a risk of TSS associated with their use. To reduce the risk, make sure to always wash your hands before and after insertion, boil your cup between periods, and have two cups in rotation. Also take care when inserting or removing your cup as abrasions on the vaginal wall can increase the risk of bacteria getting into the bloodstream.

CHOOSING A MENSTRUAL MANAGEMENT PRODUCT

Finding the best products for you isn't as overwhelming as the list above might suggest. Figure out what's comfortable and what works best for you, depending what your own period is like.

While I always recommend reusable products, I recognize that not everyone can afford the up-front cost, even if they present savings in the long run. I also recognize that accessibility is a real issue and not everyone can change a cup or even a tampon, and that there are times when the convenience of disposable products trumps all other considerations. I certainly don't pack my cloth pads when going on vacation. What you do most of the time matters more than once in a while.

Here are a few things to consider when it comes to choosing a product for managing your flow:

- **How heavy is your flow?** Always choose the lowest absorbency product, particularly for anything worn internally, and change it more often if needed to reduce the risk of toxic shock syndrome.
- **What will you be doing?** Pads, whether disposable or cloth, just aren't going to jive with a swimming pool. Think about what activities you'll be doing and where.
- **What's comfortable to wear?** Do you prefer a product that's worn internally or externally?
- **How comfortable are you with your bodily fluids?** Reusable products require a certain level of intimacy with your bodily fluids, and while I always advocate for getting up close and personal with your flow, I recognize not everyone is there, and there can be some trauma around the sight of blood.
- **What are the products made from?** When using disposable products, look for those that are 100 percent cotton and unscented. Chemicals found in rayon processing have been linked to menstrual disorders. Other products have been doused with "fragrance" to mask odours.
- **What is the environmental impact of this product?** Is it biodegradable? Do you need to throw something in the garbage bin after using it? Can it be reused? How much plastic does the product contain — both in the product and the packaging? Consider the waste of your product choices.

Check the resources section at the back of this book for a list of recommended products and where to buy them.

SLEEP

Just as you know how you feel after a healthy meal, you know how you feel after a good night's sleep. Sleep is an important piece of the period health puzzle.

Restorative, deep sleep supports hormonal health by resetting the nervous system — putting you in that juicy rest and digest state, and regulating the release of progesterone, estrogen, and luteinizing hormone (which is critical for ovulation).

Getting enough sleep can feel elusive when the days are short but prioritizing eight hours a night will have a positive effect on your hormonal health and your period. If you have difficulty falling asleep at night, start by implementing a consistent bedtime routine to transition your body and mind from the hustle and bustle of the day to relaxing to the max.

Creating a bedtime routine sounds like you're treating yourself like a toddler, but that is *exactly* what you need to do. If you've ever tried to pull a toddler away from their playroom and plunk them into bed for a nap, then you know that it's impossible for them to just curl up and fall asleep. The same is true for us grown-ups. If you've been working late or watching TV or whatever it is that you're doing that's keeping you up and out of bed, chances are you can't just hop into bed, close your eyes, and drift off to dreamland. If you're one of the few people who can, well, good on you! But if you're like most of us, you likely can't — and the reason for that is, you guessed it, hormones.

Feeling "tired but wired" at the end of the day is a hallmark sign of your adrenal glands pumping out cortisol all day and night, either because of chronic overstimulation and stress or from riding blood sugar spikes and crashes all day long (or maybe both). Making time to reset your nervous system at the end of a long day, before you jump into bed, can help make achieving a deep, restful sleep easy as pie.

Creating a Bedtime Routine

Just as with self-care and exercise, the specific steps involved in your bedtime routine aren't as important as simply having a bedtime routine. Imposing a routine is also a great way to bake in some of that scheduled self-care. Here are a few tips:

- Turn your screens off at least an hour before bedtime.
- Dim the lights.
- Take some time to unwind — have a bath or shower, light a candle (blow it out before you fall asleep!), read, whatever feels good to you.
- Create a sleep environment that is dark and cool — artificial lights interrupt sleep and hormone regulation.
- Go to bed early — you'll have better, more restorative sleep if you turn the lights out by 10:00 p.m.

VAGINAL STEAMING

If you've never heard of vaginal steaming, allow me to introduce you. It's exactly what it sounds like — imagine a steam facial, but instead of your face, you're steaming your vulva. Herbs are steeped in boiling water — just like a cup of tea — and then you sit, bottomless of course, over the pot, either on a special vaginal sauna or by simply placing the bowl or pot on the floor or in the toilet. You allow the steam to waft up to your vulva and into your vagina and subsequently the uterus.

Vaginal steaming is often cited as a treatment for irregular periods, endometriosis, dysmenorrhea, clotting, spotting, infertility, amenorrhea, fibroids, and other menstrual disorders.

I was skeptical of the practice myself — until I tried it. It was a very pleasant experience and it seemed to have a positive effect on my period, helping to restore regularity after a couple of longer-than-normal cycles.

One thing to note about the practice is that vaginal steaming isn't used for "cleaning" the vagina — something that you don't actually need to do, as your vagina is equipped with its own mechanisms for housekeeping. The healing properties found in the herbs used for vaginal steaming are thought to support and tone the vulva, vagina, and uterus, which can help to clear up menstrual discomfort or disorders.

And while the cervix does help to keep the uterus sealed when the os is closed, steam is actually a pretty powerful substance. Keli Garza is the founder of Steamy Chick, a company that distributes vaginal saunas and herbs and trains vaginal stream facilitators. She points out that steam has the power to permeate rock — so surely it can make it past a cervix.

Depending on which symptoms you're trying to treat, herbs used in vaginal steams may include rosemary, lavender, oregano, marigold, basil, chamomile, rose petals, parsley, red clover, burdock leaf, or motherwort. Many spas offer the service in house, and vaginal steam packets, which look like oversized tea bags, are available online from many retailers.

Vaginal steaming should be avoided during pregnancy, when you're menstruating, and after ovulation if you're trying to achieve pregnancy. And of course, take the necessary precautions to avoid burns. Test the steam with the underside of your wrist before sitting down. If steam ever feels too hot, stand up for a few minutes to let it cool before sitting back down.

CASTOR OIL PACKS

Another favourite naturopathic or traditional remedy is a castor oil pack. Castor oil comes from the *Ricinus communis*, or castor oil plant. Its healing properties are believed to come from the high concentration of ricinoleic acid contained in the oil. Used topically, it can help to stimulate circulation, liver function, and the lymphatic system, which is an important part of your immune function. Castor oil packs can be helpful for cramps, fibroids, cysts, endometriosis, adenomyosis, PMS, and other issues related to estrogen dominance, such as a heavy flow.

Castor oil packs can be applied to the abdomen for cramping, cysts, or fibroids, or on the upper right quadrant of the abdomen from the midline around to the back to stimulate the liver, which can help promote hormone balance.

Here are two ways to reap the benefits of castor oil:

- Option 1: Soak a clean piece of flannel or cotton (you can use an old t-shirt) with castor oil. Place fabric on the body, cover with water-resistant fabric like oilcloth or nylon (or you can reuse a plastic shopping bag) to keep the oil on your skin and off everything else, and apply a hot water bottle or heat pack. Relax for twenty to thirty minutes. Rinse off any castor oil that may have got on your skin. Store castor-soaked fabric in the fridge.
- Option 2: Apply castor oil directly to your skin. Apply heat (optional). Relax for twenty to thirty minutes. Rinse castor oil from your skin.

Be aware that castor oil will stain fabric, so be warned before wearing your favourite clothes or using your best towels when using castor oil packs.

RECOMMENDATIONS FOR
SPECIFIC PERIOD PROBLEMS

While the aforementioned guidelines should be helpful for any and all menstrual-related disorders, there are a few things to focus on if you are experiencing a specific issue related to your period. Here's what changes to focus on making based on the problem you may be experiencing.

Acne	Avoid dairy products Identify food sensitivities Support digestion Do a gentle liver detox
Amenorrhea	Lower stress to reduce cortisol Support the thyroid Use seed cycling to balance hormones Ensure you're getting enough calories and nutrients Promote ovulation
Breast tenderness/pain	Avoid caffeine Use seed cycling to balance hormones Avoid soy
Cysts	Regulate blood sugar Use castor oil packs
Endometriosis	Support anti-inflammation Avoid gluten Identify food sensitivities
Heavy periods	Reduce estrogen Support digestion Avoid soy
Painful periods	Support anti-inflammation Reduce estrogen
PCOS	Regulate blood sugar Support the thyroid

CHAPTER 11

MANAGING YOUR PERIOD PAIN

One thing to remember when it comes to dietary changes for period pain is that it's a marathon, not a sprint. You can't start eating anti-inflammatory, hormone-supporting foods when you're in your PMS window or on day one of your cycle and expect to reap the benefits right away. You can't isolate your period from the rest of your menstrual cycle, and so you need to be supporting your hormonal and menstrual health every day of the month. It takes one hundred days for the follicles in your ovaries to release an egg at ovulation. So, your diet and nutrition need to support all one hundred days of their journey.

Some light cramping and fatigue are considered normal in the days leading up to and during your period. And even if you're making all the right changes to your diet and lowering your stress levels and toxic load, there might be a time when you still experience some pain and discomfort. While ibuprofen is known to lower prostaglandins and therefore ease cramps, headaches, and other types of pain, it also comes with risks to your heart, bone, and kidney health, as well as your hearing. Frequent use of ibuprofen more than doubles your risk of a major heart event.[1]

Here are a few ways that you can manage acute pain related to menstruation in the long and short term.

Diet
Changing your diet to one that is anti-inflammatory and based on whole, unprocessed foods is the front-line response to combatting period pain without the use of hormonal birth control or painkillers. Eliminating foods

that are known to cause inflammation, such as sugar, alcohol, caffeine, and processed and packaged foods, can help to lower your overall inflammation and reduce prostaglandins. Cutting out any foods that you may be sensitive or allergic to is also key. Refer to the nutrition section of this book for more on changing your diet.

Magnesium

Magnesium is an essential nutrient for all-around hormonal health, supporting the nervous system, blood sugar regulation, promoting sleep, and more. Dietary sources include dark chocolate, green leafy vegetables, and salmon. But it is especially helpful as a supplement when it comes to period pain because it works as a muscle relaxant, calming uterine contractions. It is also helpful for headaches and migraines that might appear in the days leading up to and during menstruation. Look for powdered magnesium citrate or bisglycinate, which can be mixed with hot water for a warm, relaxing beverage before bed.

Physical Therapies

The physical positioning of our uterus in our bodies can contribute to period pain. If it's tilted back or forward, it can inhibit the efficiency of uterine contractions to shed the lining during menstruation. If the uterus has to work harder to shed the lining and work it out through the cervix and into the vagina, your period will be more painful. Scarring from endometriosis or a Caesarean birth can also increase pain. Physical therapies such as pelvic floor physiotherapy or abdominal massage can help to reposition the uterus in a more efficient way within the body, which may alleviate menstrual cramps, and help break up scar tissue or adhesions.

Cannabis and CBD

While research is lacking when it comes to how pot interacts specifically with periods or the reproductive system, there is solid evidence that cannabis relieves pain.[2] Anecdotally, there is no shortage of people using cannabis to treat menstrual-related symptoms. Maya Elizabeth, co-founder of Whoopi & Maya, a California-based company that produces typical cannabis products to relieve menstrual pain, describes cannabis as having always been a "woman's ally."[3] References to cannabis being used for menstrual pain go all the way back to the 1500s when a Chinese medical textbook recommended cannabis flowers to ease symptoms during menstruation. Even Queen Victoria reportedly used cannabis each month!

As Canada and some U.S. states move to legalize medical and recreational use of cannabis, there's no shortage of products hitting the market that are geared toward PMS and menstrual pain. Besides good old-fashioned weed for smoking, you can now get topical creams, bath bombs, edibles, oils, tinctures, and even vaginal suppositories to alleviate your cramps, menstrual migraines, and other PMS symptoms. Not all products contain THC, the psychoactive ingredient in cannabis that makes you feel high. Cannabidiol, known as CBD, is the compound in cannabis that has the medical benefits but doesn't have a psychoactive effect.

If you're going to try cannabis for menstrual pain, look for a reputable source that sells a high-quality version of CBD, and of course be mindful of laws and regulations where you live before purchasing cannabis.

TENS (Transcutaneous Electrical Nerve Stimulation)

TENS uses electric currents to stimulate nerves and reduce pain. In trials it has been shown to ease menstrual pain, lessen the frequency of ibuprofen use, and significantly reduce diarrhea, menstrual flow, clot formation, and fatigue.[4] To use a TENS machine, electrodes are placed over the pain site using stick-on pads. Then you simply turn it on. When in use it feels like a gentle vibration. TENS is also used in labour and for the relief of other types of pain. Consumer units are priced from as low as fifty dollars and are easy and safe to use, with no known side effects.

Yoga

Yoga can be a great way to relieve menstrual pain or to get some movement in during a time when you might have lower energy or fatigue. There are several yoga poses that can help to relieve menstrual pain, including the child's pose (resting on your knees with your forehead on the ground) and butterfly (reclining on your back with your feet together and knees apart).

Restorative forms of yoga that hold poses longer, using props like bolsters and cushions for support, can be particularly enjoyable when you're tired or crampy.

Some yoga teachers suggest avoiding inversions during menstruation to keep your energy flowing down and out. Talk to your instructor about modifications based on how you're feeling that day — as always, it's best to listen to your body.

Orgasms

Having an orgasm can help to relieve the pain of menstrual cramps thanks to the dopamine, oxytocin, and endorphins that are released with a climax. All three are known to relieve pain.

Get down with a partner — or on your own if you're not feeling amorous. Concerned about the mess? Throw down a towel or use a menstrual management product that's worn internally to contain your flow.

Herbs and Botanical Medicine

There are a number of herbs and botanical plant medicines that are often prescribed to alleviate menstrual pain, including crampbark, vitex, and red raspberry leaf. Herbal remedies come as teas, capsules or tablets, tinctures (liquid extracts), or steams.

Something to remember is that herbs and plants are medicine — you wouldn't walk into a pharmacy and just take any bottle down off the shelf. The same goes for botanicals. Get your herbs from a reputable source and talk to someone who is qualified to help you find the correct herb, dosage, and format.

CHAPTER 12

HORMONAL HEALTH AFTER BIRTH CONTROL

COMING OFF THE PILL

Whether you're stopping in order to get pregnant or because it's simply not working for you any longer, deciding to stop taking hormonal contraception is a big decision and can feel like a daunting task, regardless of how long you've been on it. If you originally started taking hormonal birth control because of bad periods — painful cramping, irregular periods, acne, or any of the symptoms that are commonly treated with hormonal contraception — it can be scary to think about the pain and discomfort that might be waiting for you on the other side once you stop taking it.

While there's no way to tell what your periods are going to be like when you stop taking hormonal birth control — for better or for worse, it might be the same, it might not be — the age that you started taking hormones, what your periods were like before you started, and your individual body makeup might give you an indication.

Be prepared for anything. You may have an easy time, or you may not. If you're currently taking hormonal contraception and want to conceive, give yourself lots of time to get your cycles back in order before you start trying. Having a difficult transition off of hormonal birth control can be especially overwhelming if you're stopping with the hopes of becoming pregnant. When the stakes are high, it's easy to feel discouraged with absent periods or irregular cycles. Try to stay focused on the end goal — not just fertility, but your overall health and wellness. And if your cycles return before you're ready to start trying make sure you have a non-homonal birth control plan in place.

Below are some guidelines for transitioning off the pill or other forms of hormonal contraception.

Commit

One of the things that kept me on hormonal birth control for so long was frustration with irregular periods, long cycles, and symptoms like heavy bleeding and cramping. It was just easier to go back on the pill. But if you've decided that the pill no longer aligns with your values, you're experiencing side effects, or you're trying to become pregnant, then you need to commit to the process of transitioning off of birth control and supporting your health.

Learn How to Chart

Coming off of hormonal contraception is a great time to learn menstrual cycle awareness. Learn how to chart your menstrual cycle and how to interpret the signs of fertility. Charting during your transition can help you to pinpoint any hormonal imbalances that may have cropped up as a result of the pill, or nutrient deficiencies that might be having a downstream effect on your hormones. It will also help you to get back in touch with the natural ebbs and flows that you will likely feel as the flat-line of synthetic hormones is replaced with the ups and downs of progesterone and estrogen.

Be Prepared with Alternate Contraception

If you're coming off hormonal birth control but still want to avoid pregnancy, you're going to need to have an alternative form of contraception at the ready for those times when you want to have penis-ejaculating-in-vagina sex around your fertile window. Remember that you will ovulate before you get your first post-pill period, after the withdrawal bleed you'll experience when you stop taking hormonal contraception. In other words, you'll hit a fertile phase before you get your first period, so plan accordingly.

Condoms are always a good option with a high efficacy rate. Cervical caps and diaphragms are also options.

If you're planning to use a Fertility Awareness Method as a form of contraception, I recommend working with a qualified holistic reproductive health practitioner or Fertility Awareness Educator who can teach you the ins and outs of charting, help you interpret your chart, and determine your fertile window so you know when you are safe from pregnancy and when you're at risk.

Keep a Journal

You may want to keep a journal to note any symptoms or changes as you are transitioning off of hormonal birth control. It can be particularly interesting to overlay what you record in your journal with your menstrual awareness chart to get in touch with how your hormones influence other factors in your life.

NUTRITIONAL SUPPORT POST-BIRTH CONTROL

Hormonal contraceptives cause more nutrient deficiencies than any other prescription drug.[1] Functional medicine and holistic health practitioners are even recognizing a collection of symptoms caused by the nutritional deficiencies of hormonal contraceptives, called Post-Pill Syndrome. Symptoms may include a complete loss of menstruation, hypothyroidism, headaches, depression, anxiety, or digestive issues.[2] Therefore, if you decide to use hormonal contraceptives, it is important that you support your body with good nutrition to make up for what's lost.

Here are a few key things to consider from a nutritional standpoint, either while you are taking hormonal birth control or transitioning off of it.

Because it's likely that you will be deficient in one or more vitamins or minerals after taking hormonal contraception, this is one of those times that I believe there is a benefit to taking high-quality supplements. Purchase the highest quality supplements that you can afford, and work with a qualified nutritionist or naturopath to help you choose the right dosage based on your own personal needs.

B Vitamins

Hormonal contraception can deplete a number of B vitamins, including B2, B6, B9, and B12. While we need all our B vitamins, of course, these particular B vitamins also happen to be essential for hormonal health. B9, in particular, also known as folate, is a critical supplement pre- and post-conception, as a lack of folate is known to contribute to birth defects. B vitamins work together, so take a good quality B-complex vitamin that contains a balanced level of each type of B vitamin. If you are deficient in a particular B vitamin — for instance, many of us require extra B5, our stress B vitamin — you can take a B complex in addition to a stand-alone

B supplement to make sure that you're getting what you need. Taking a B vitamin on its own can throw your other B vitamins out of balance.

Probiotics

Long-term use of hormonal contraception can wreak havoc on our gut health and microbiome, so it's important to eat a small serving of fermented foods every day. It's also a good idea to supplement with a good quality probiotic that contains at least two or three different strains, and a minimum of 10 billion CFU per the daily recommendation.

Zinc

Another essential nutrient for hormonal health and, in particular, fertility, zinc can be depleted by hormonal birth control.

Magnesium

Magnesium helps to regulate blood sugar, supports the nervous system, and chills us out.

Multivitamins and Minerals

I'm not always a fan of recommending multivitamins and minerals, but given that the list of nutrients depleted by hormonal birth control is so long, it can be helpful when you're coming off it. Take a good-quality, full-spectrum multivitamin that includes minerals as well as vitamins. Even if you're not planning on conceiving, many prenatal vitamins are specially formulated with the nutrients you need to support hormonal health and fertility. Look for a brand that doesn't include a lot of filler, which may include soy, gluten, corn, and other commonly irritating foods.

◆ PART 3 ◆
EMBRACING YOUR CYCLE

CHAPTER 13
TUNING IN TO YOUR CYCLE

> How much power is in a woman's menstrual blood? How much power is in a woman's menstrual cycle? The power to create life is in our menstrual cycle and here we are thinking our periods are dirty and gross, and thinking there's something wrong with us because we bleed when that's where every single human being has come from. What if we really knew how powerful we really are?
> — Lisa Hendrickson-Jack, *Heavy Flow* podcast

If the shame of menstruation is born from misogynistic attitudes and teachings rather than facts, then perhaps it's also true that the negative attitudes towards menstruation and the menstrual cycle — that it's a curse, something that is inconvenient and valuable only if we wish to have a child, and then something to wait out until menopause — have also been taught.

Can we improve our experience of our menstrual cycles simply by changing our minds about it?

Much of what we in the industrialized world have been taught about menstruation was shaped not just by corporations that have a financial interest in your shame and taboo, but by *people who don't even menstruate*. Men have been writing about and theorizing about menstruation since the dawn of time, it seems. And getting it dead wrong, I might add.

A survey that looked at the development of menstrual-related beliefs and behaviours in adolescence noted that girls who learned more about menstruation from male sources rated menstruation as more debilitating and negative than those who learned less from male sources.[1]

Menstruation is rarely, if ever, framed in a positive light in the media or in product marketing. Social scientists have long documented negative attitudes toward menstruation and how it affects our experience. These negative attitudes may play a role in shaping our experiences of menstruation, as well as promoting ignorance about this vital bodily function.

Many people of all genders are unable to describe the process of the menstrual cycle and may be confused about the hormones and organs involved. Hell, many people don't even know the correct name for the external female genitalia, incorrectly referring to the vulva as a vagina.

There appears to be some evidence that reframing menstruation as a positive experience is enough to change our perception of the experience.

In the late 1960s, the Menstrual Distress Questionnaire was developed (by a man) as a standardized method for collecting data about menstrual cycle symptoms. The survey asked respondents to rate their experiences of forty-seven different symptoms that occurred before and during menstruation on a six-point scale. Ratings ranged from no symptoms to acute or partially disabling. The survey didn't even allow for reporting positive aspects of menstruation; respondents were only able to respond negatively to menstrual experiences.

In 1987, the authors of *The Curse: A Cultural History of Menstruation* developed the Menstrual Joy Questionnaire to test the theory that reframing menstruation positively could change a menstruator's perceptions of their period experience. The questionnaire asked respondents to report the positive effects of menstruation, like heightened creativity and increased sexual libido. Those who completed the questionnaire a week before they completed the Menstrual Distress Questionnaire reported fewer negative symptoms. While subsequent attempts to recreate the Menstrual Joy Questionnaire didn't turn up quite the same results, these findings do reflect what I have heard anecdotally.

The number one thing that I hear from listeners of the *Heavy Flow* podcast and those who attend my workshops is that they had never considered their period to be anything other than a negative experience until they understood the importance of menstruation as a vital sign. Everything that they had been taught about menstruation up until that point skewed negative; it never occurred to them that menstruation could be anything but a curse. Learning the concept of body literacy and recognizing the value in the menstrual cycle can be a life-altering kind of moment. Once you start to recognize the patterns of your menstrual cycle and hormones, it's hard to turn away from that knowledge.

There's something to be said for the power of persuasion.

My hope is that this book will give you the tools to understand and embrace your cycle in the way that is most meaningful to *you*. That might mean going full-on moon goddess or getting to the last page and never giving your menstrual cycle another thought. Or maybe, like me, you'll fall somewhere in the middle (and even then, my attitude and approach to my cycle is fluid).

When I was preparing for pregnancy, I was laser focused on charting to know exactly when I was fertile and adding fertility-boosting foods to my diet. While writing this book, I looked at my cycle with a sense of wonder — it was amazing to see all of the research and knowledge that I had collected over the years playing out in my own cycle. Then there was the week I got my period on our family vacation and I didn't give it a second thought.

So, no matter how — or *if* — you choose to embrace your cycle, it's all good. What works for you will change over time.

CHAPTER 14

WORKING WITH, NOT AGAINST, YOUR HORMONES

Thanks to our hormones, our bodies, like nature, are cyclical, and you shouldn't expect yourself to feel the same 24/7/365 — because you won't. Unfortunately, we live in a society that values sameness and productivity.

"Being hormonal" is often used as an insult to suggest that a woman is being irrational, overly emotional, or is unfit for a particular job. This attitude is just another instrument of the patriarchy designed to keep female bodies "othered" and oppressed. But your hormonal cycles offer an opportunity to tune in and use them to your advantage.

Your hormones do more than just turn you on or give you PMS. Hormones play a role in every bodily process, affecting everything from your menstrual cycles to your moods, appetite, sleep patterns, and much, much more.

When you start to tune in to your menstrual cycle and observe the different phases of your cycle, you may start to notice that there is a natural rise and fall to your energy, creativity, and focus — certain times of your cycle where you might feel more energetic, clear-headed, and productive (I like to call this the Beyoncé phase), and other times when you feel like your head is in the clouds, you're dragging your feet, and it's impossible to get anything done. Instead of fighting against these ebbs and flows, it's possible to use them to your advantage.[1]

The practice of organizing your life in accordance to the hormonal shifts of your menstrual cycle is often referred to as "life cycling." It can be as simple as recognizing where you are in your cycle and taking note of your mood or energy. Or you can use your menstrual cycle to guide scheduling certain personal, social, or business activities in order to maximize the effects of your hormonal ebb and flow. This might look like choosing restorative yoga over spinning when your energy is lower; or perhaps scheduling a social engagement for the peak of your follicular phase, when rising estrogen levels are likely to make you feel chattier and more sociable.

Of course, I recognize that the practice of life cycling isn't accessible to everyone all the time, and I know there is a certain privilege inherent in the concept of life cycling or even "embracing" menstruation at all. If you work, or care for young children, or especially if you do both, taking a few days off to rest while you're on your period isn't going to be possible for most people. Not everyone can rest when they need to rest. Not everyone can choose to say no because their cycles don't align with the required energy levels or moods with a certain activity.

At the very least, understanding how your menstrual cycle affects your physical health and tuning in to it can assure you that it's not all just in your head — there really are days of the month or of your cycle when your energy levels or your mood are higher or lower. So much of the female experience is being told that things are all in your head, and so understanding your hormone cycles and recognizing how they unfold in your own life can be vindicating … and empowering.

When you no longer expect to feel the same way every single day, a new world cracks wide open. There are days when you're going to feel more ambitious and days when you're going to feel more cautious, turning inward. Being able to honour where you're at and give your body what it needs, when possible, can be incredibly powerful and have a profound effect on your health. But if you ignore what your body is telling you when it's whispering, you'll have no choice but to listen when it starts to yell.

HOW YOUR HORMONES AFFECT YOUR LIFE: PHASE TO PHASE

Hormones are at work in every cell in your body, and as they fluctuate throughout your menstrual cycle, so do your moods, energy levels, and so much more. When you start to track your menstrual cycle, you can also take note of how much energy you have, your sex drive, your appetite, your food cravings — anything that may change from day to day. Before long, you may start to see patterns emerging.

Here is a look at how the hormones at play in each phase of your menstrual cycle might have an influence on other factors in your life. Of course, we are all different, and hormones aren't the be-all and end-all of how we experience and perceive our lives, so you don't have to check every single box in every single phase in order to be "normal."

For a refresher on the hormones and phases of the menstrual cycle, be sure to take a look back at the chapter on the physiology of menstrual cycles.

The cyclical nature of the menstrual cycle in some ways mirrors the cycles of nature and the seasons. Some people find it helpful to align the various phases of the menstrual cycle with the seasons, not just as a way to tune in and understand what's happening in each phase, but also to form a connection between an individual and nature and the environment. In the same way that we cycle throughout the phases of our menstrual cycle, the earth cycles through the four seasons — winter, spring, summer, and fall.

Menstruation — Day 1

Energy may be low, and your body is preparing for a new cycle. Both ovarian and gonadotropin hormones start out low at the onset of a new menstrual cycle. During menstruation, you may still experience pain from cramping, or other symptoms, which may have an effect on your mood.

A NOTE ABOUT TRACKING

Self-observation is interesting to some and boring to others; I don't mean to suggest that we should be tracking all this data on ourselves at all times. I know from personal experience that tracking your menstrual cycles, body temperature, food, exercise, and other factors all at once can be exhausting and, at times, trigger anxiety and obsessive behaviours. I suggest tracking for a few months in order to establish your baseline and learn your "normal," so you can start to see the patterns emerging. But if tracking and charting isn't something that you're particularly fond of, or you find that you are becoming obsessive or stressed about it, by all means, stop. There are more important things in life than tracking your periods. The one exception to this rule is if you are looking to use a Fertility Awareness Method of birth control. In that case, charting your cycle daily is essential.

Your period, the week or so of your cycle when you are menstruating, is aligned with the winter. This is a time of inward reflection and of metaphorical death as the endometrium is shed from the uterus.

The Follicular Phase

As estrogen rises during the first half of your cycle, so does mood and energy; you may start to feel more energetic, chattier, and more willing to take risks. Gabrielle Lichterman, founder of Hormonology, describes this phase as going "upwards and outwards." Aligned with the fresh energy of spring, your follicular phase is when you're likely feeling your best; you wake up in a good mood feeling like everything in life is great!

During this time, you might feel you want to get out of the house more, to socialize and meet new people. That's not a mistake — there is an evolutionary advantage to wanting to get out of the house and into the world as you're approaching ovulation. Sex drives surge during this phase, peaking around ovulation.

This is also a great time for those activities that require more energy and enthusiasm. As we naturally start to crave healthier foods during this phase, it's a good time to start implementing some of the changes discussed in the nutrition section of this book — they are more likely to become lasting habits when we work with our natural inclination for healthier foods in the follicular phase.

Life seems filled with possibilities in the spring months, and this is what the follicular phase feels like, too. Our energy is high, and we feel ready to take on the world. This is a time of rebirth and renewal as we begin a new cycle.

Ovulation

At the point in your menstrual cycle when the egg is released from the follicle, some people report feeling energetic, while others say that this is when they start to turn inward as their energy spirals downward. If you are sensitive to the dramatic hormonal shifts that take place during ovulation, you may experience symptoms around this time. Your sex drive generally peaks just before or at ovulation, which makes sense because if you are trying to conceive you'll need to be in the mood.

As we approach ovulation, our bodies are in full bloom, as in summer. When the sun is shining and plants are in full bloom, the world feels lush and plush, and your body may, too.

The Luteal Phase

This final phase of your menstrual cycle is when progesterone is produced — after the egg is released from the follicle of the ovary, the corpus luteum manufactures progesterone. Thanks to that progesterone, you may feel that your energy has dropped and find yourself opting to stay closer to home. During this phase you may feel more introspective and turn your focus inward. Think about the last time you cancelled plans to stay home and watch Netflix by yourself; could you have been in your luteal phase?

You might start to crave higher fat, higher calorie foods during this phase, because progesterone is responsible for sustaining and nourishing a pregnancy. It makes sense, then, that you would start to crave these foods at this time.

Once we have ovulated and summer's brightness comes to a close, we enter autumn. Now our body is preparing for the long winter. Hormones dip, and we may start to feel symptoms of PMS as we approach menstruation.

GOING DEEPER: FINDING MEANING OR SPIRITUAL CONNECTION

Those early medical scholars I mentioned in the introduction, who wrote about menstruation as a powerful force: what if they were onto something? Could it be that there really is some magic, mysticism, or power inherent in menstrual blood and the act of menstruation?

As with all aspects of embracing your menstrual cycle, it's up to you to decide. But many people who menstruate find that the time leading up to and during menstruation is a period (pun intended) of increased spiritual connection, even psychic ability. Many people report dreams that are more vivid or creative.

The energy of the menstrual cycle is what Alexandra Pope and Sjanie Hugo Wurlitzer describe as "wild power." Others might refer to it as "womb wisdom" or the more gendered and familiar term "women's intuition."

Whatever you want to call it, there is potential to assign spiritual meaning and connection to your menstrual cycle if that resonates with you.

From the earliest writings about menstruation, people have associated it with creative energy. It's an in-between state, an outward symbol of fertility, yet also a symbol that no baby has been created. It is, at once, a symbol of life and death.

Is this creative energy something that can only be applied to the creation of a new human life? If you're not interested in becoming pregnant during a given cycle — or ever — does that mean that this energy is not available to you, or that it is lost?

Samantha Zipporah, who describes herself as a "practical and radical medicine woman," believes that we can all tap into the creative energy of the menstrual cycle, regardless of our desire to reproduce. This creative energy can be applied to artistic endeavours, business ventures, or other aspects of life. When you choose to say no to a pregnancy — either because you're using contraception, or you've chosen to have an abortion — you're not just saying no to having a baby; you're saying yes to something else.

"You're not avoiding or ending a pregnancy for no reason at all," Zipporah says. "You're doing that because there is something you want to engage your vital life force in that is not gestating, birthing, and raising a human child. There is profound medicine in claiming the sacred yes."

So, how do you harness this creative energy? Just as we must find our own way to relate to our menstrual cycles, the same holds true for finding a deeper meaning or spiritual connection within your menstrual cycle.

Certainly, not every culture from the dawn of time looked at the menstrual cycle as something shameful and disgusting; there is plenty to be read about various times and places where the menstruating woman has been celebrated, even revered. It should come as no shock when I tell you that these societies generally didn't adhere to the patriarchal ideologies that dominate much of the Western world. One place to look is in traditional teachings or histories of your own culture. You might find rituals or rites that are associated with menarche, monthly menstruation, or even menopause.

While I encourage you to find the ways of celebrating your menstrual cycle that feel natural to you, always be mindful of cultural appropriation.

CHAPTER 15
TALKING TO THE NEXT GENERATION

As a parent, I recognize that the future of the world rests in the hands of my daughter and her peers. It's not enough for us to be period positive now; we need to raise the next generation of menstruators to be truly free of shame and allow them to define their relationship with their menstrual cycles on their own terms.

Talking to the next generation about menstruation first involves being comfortable with this bodily function yourself. If you are shackled in shame and taboo, how will you ever talk confidently and appropriately to younger people about it? Understand how your menstrual cycle works and why it's important, not just to your fertility, but to your overall health and wellness. Think about your own relationship to your menstrual cycle and how that shows up for you month to month. Having a solid understanding and foundation ourselves is the key to passing on period positivity.

In the same way that body shame and diet culture is passed down from one generation to the next, so, too, is period shame. Children are sponges who soak up everything they see and hear from us, including that passive remark about your gross, annoying period. Try not to make disparaging remarks or jokes about menstruation when children and adolescents are within earshot. Even if you think they're not listening, they absorb this information.

Instead, make menstruation a normal, neutral part of everyday life. When children are young it's impossible to use the washroom without them barging in or insisting on accompanying you to the toilet. If you're menstruating and changing a pad or tampon, or emptying a cup, use this as a time to be frank and honest with them about what is happening using age-appropriate language. If you're open with them about what is happening in your body, what you are doing to care for yourself, and why it's an important facet of health and wellness, it will help to normalize menstruation when they encounter it themselves — when they are learning about menstrual cycles in health class, talking to a doctor about their own experience, or supporting a friend or loved one who is menstruating.

While it's impossible to untangle the menstrual cycle from its reproductive function, it's essential that we don't reduce it to that. Yes, it's true that when an adolescent girl reaches menarche she becomes fertile and can have a baby, but it's important that we don't use this fact as a way to scare her. Adolescence is a confusing time, and young people receive a lot of mixed messages — particularly when it comes to their bodies. Of course, menarche is an opportunity to talk with girls about sex, fertility, birth control, STIs, and other important topics that need to be broached, but simply focusing on the fact that she can now have a baby and using that to scare her is going to do more harm than good.

We must also be careful that the conversation about menstruation doesn't centre solely on products and menstrual management. Yes, of course this is the time to teach a young person how to properly use a pad, tampon, or cup — hygiene is important — but it's also a good time to tell her about the other exciting things that happen when you're a teenager going through puberty.

Laura Wershler, a veteran sexual and reproductive health advocate, cautions against simply telling adolescents that when they get their period, they can get pregnant. This is an opportunity to instill knowledge and power. Help them understand that getting their periods is going to make them stronger, more capable, and more creative, and that there's a responsibility that comes with that change — the responsibility to manage our fertility and sexual health. Framing the menstrual cycle as a vital sign important to our overall health and wellness means that we're not treating our fertility like an enemy that we have to control until we, maybe someday, want to take advantage of it. Fertility is a friend to our health and well-being at all times.

As a society, we are becoming more aware of issues around gender and are recognizing that not everyone identifies with traditional gender binaries. Because of this, I caution against language that frames menstruation as "what makes you a woman" — regardless of how you assume your child might identify on the gender spectrum. Your period isn't what makes you a woman at all. There are plenty of women who do not menstruate — because of menopause, health conditions, or menstrual suppression via hormonal birth control. Are they less of a woman because they don't or may never have menstruated? There are also plenty of trans men and non-binary folks who menstruate, but do not identify as a woman. Gender is much more nuanced than simply getting your period, and we should be sensitive to that when discussing menstruation, not just with young people, but at all times.

It is confusing to announce to a young girl that she is a woman now that she has started her period, only to then unleash an avalanche of shame, taboo, and consumerism. *You are a woman now, but it's going to suck because now you'll get cramps and also nobody must know. You must ensure that no one ever sees or hears that your body is menstruating.* That type of rhetoric is confusing and is only compounded with the mixed messages of sexuality that girls are also receiving at this age.

In fact, the menstrual taboo can increase self-sexualization and objectification. Because the menstrual taboo makes young people want to hide their bleeding, they may instead highlight their sexual bodies as a way to suppress their menstruating ones.[1]

Education around menstrual cycles, puberty, and sexual health that is free from corporate interest is also essential. Say no to the pamphlets and online websites that are produced by corporations using shame and taboo to sell their products. Instead, look for books, websites, and other forms of content that are independently produced and don't attempt to sell you solutions to problems that don't really exist.

Raising period-positive kids — of all sexes and gender identities — is the key to freeing us *all* from shame and taboo. Young children who grow up in a household where menstruation is normalized will be more comfortable with menstruation when they reach puberty. Understanding the menstrual cycle as a vital sign, beyond fertility, may also positively influence how young people make decisions around sex and birth control, and may help them preserve their fertility when the time comes.

And who knows: some of these young children who grow up understanding that menstrual cycles are an essential, vital sign may grow up to become doctors, researchers, and other medical professionals who can help to eradicate the gender bias that keeps menstruators suffering from the pain of menstruation.

CONCLUSION

The cure for the curse of menstruation, according to Elizabeth Kissling, author of *Capitalizing on the Curse: The Business of Menstruation*, is to learn to relate to your menstrual cycle on your own terms. If the menstrual taboo is shaped by cultural attitudes and big business, then the curse of menstrual shame and stigma can be broken. Each of us who menstruates has the power to break that curse in our hands.

If the ultimate goal of menstrual justice is for each of us to define our own menstrual experience, in our own way, then that means that there is no singular or correct way to "embrace" your menstrual cycle.

Unfortunately, that also means that I don't have a neat little checklist that I can plug in to the end of this book to help you figure out how to relate to your own menstrual cycle. If we are to free ourselves of the shackles that have come from centuries of shame, taboo, and misunderstanding, we must find out what our menstrual cycles mean to us individually.

My hope is that in this book, I've framed your menstrual cycle and your period in a new way for you. Once you understand the role of the menstrual cycle as a vital sign, beyond fertility, and you start to feel relief from menstrual-related symptoms, perhaps you'll begin to feel that maybe it's not such a curse after all.

It's time for menstruators to define our own menstrual experience — as women, as trans men, as non-binary people, and everyone in between.

ACKNOWLEDGEMENTS

This project is not mine alone. There are many people to whom I owe deep gratitude and love.

First and foremost, thank you to the menstrual activists, women's health advocates, and feminists that have come before me. Your hard work and dedication have paved the way for me to do this work.

Thank you to the guests, listeners, and partners of the *Heavy Flow* podcast — without you this book would not have been possible. Thank you also to the ladies of Smashtermind for supporting the podcast from the moment I blurted out that I was going to launch a podcast. And to Rachel Laird, for *Heavy Flow*'s creative direction and graphic design, and just being the best all-around sister I could ask for.

Thank you to Margaret Bryant for affirming what I have sensed since I was just a girl — as it turns out, yes, I did have a book in me (maybe more than one!). Thank you to Allison Hirst and Heather Bean for coaxing an even better book out of me. And to the team at Dundurn Press for bringing this book into the world.

Thank you to Ashleigh Gardner for being by my side through this process and every other life event that's ever mattered.

Jenna Kalinsky, you were a most patient and supportive book doula, helping me breathe through the contractions of writing this book. You were the first one to convince me that I really could do this. Thank you.

Thank you to Emily Rose Antflick, Amy Sutherland, Laura Wershler, Lindsay Zier-Vogel, and the Semi-Retired Hens for your generous and thoughtful feedback on early drafts.

Thanks to Chris Bobel for being so generous with your time and support, and for welcoming me into the Menstruati fold.

Thank you to Angie Richards, my blue rose, for always being there, even when "there" is on the opposite side of the globe.

Thanks to Deborah Mesher for being my number one fan. You make me feel brave.

Alison Pearce, see you at our table.

To my cycle sister, Jana Girdauskas, thank you for cheering me across the finish line of writing this manuscript.

Thank you to Alex Smith-Plasterer and Amanda Gelfant for being the ones that *I* text when my period is being weird. Your friendship makes motherhood better.

To my parents, Jim and Kathleen, and to my family, thank you for a lifetime of love and support. When you told me I could be or do anything I'm sure "menstrual mogul" was not what you had in mind.

Last, and certainly not least, thank you to Jeff for being an equal parent, for always taking out the recycling, and for all the other acts of service you do that leave me to do crazy things like start podcasts and write books. I love you. And to Maisie Clementine, sweet little baby of mine, for bringing your bright light into my world.

RESOURCES

In this section you will find a list of resources, approved by *Heavy Flow*, to help you break the curse of menstruation. From products that are safe and environmentally friendly, to sources of information about the serious diseases of menstruation — you'll find it here.

FERTILITY AND MENSTRUAL CYCLE AWARENESS

Association of Fertility Awareness Professionals:
    fertilityawarenessprofessionals.com
Daysy: daysy.me
Fertility Friday: fertilityfriday.com
The Fifth Vital Sign: 5thvitalsign.com
Justisse Healthworks for Women: justisse.ca
Taking Charge of Your Fertility: tcoyf.com

MENSTRUAL CYCLE AWARENESS APPS

Clue: helloclue.com
Hormonology: myhormonology.com
Kindara: kindara.com

MENSTRUAL ACTIVISM AND ADVOCACY

Bleeding While Trans: bleedingwhiletrans.com
Menstrual Hygiene Day: menstrualhygieneday.org
Period Equity: periodequity.org

RESEARCH AND EDUCATION

Centre for Menstrual Cycle and Ovulation Research (CeMCOR):
 cemcor.ubc.ca
Cycles and Sex: cyclesandsex.com
Harlot (ad-free sex and reproductive health education for teens):
 callmeharlot.com
Menstrual Matters: menstrual-matters.com
The Society for Menstrual Cycle Research: menstruationresearch.org

ENDOMETRIOSIS EDUCATION, AWARENESS, AND SUPPORT

The Endometriosis Network Canada: endometriosisnetwork.com
Endometriosis Foundation of America: endofound.org
Know Your Endo: knowyourendo.com
Bad Periods: badperiods.com

POLYCYSTIC OVARIAN SYNDROME (PCOS) EDUCATION, AWARENESS, AND SUPPORT

Androgen Excess and PCOS Society: ae-society.org
PCOS Awareness Foundation: pcosaa.org
PCOS Diva: pcosdiva.com

PERIOD MANAGEMENT PRODUCTS

Lunapads (cloth pads, period underwear, and online retailer of the
 DivaCup): lunapads.com
Panty Prop (affordable period underwear and bathing suits):
 pantyprop.com

Glad Rags (eco-friendly pads and menstrual cups): gladrags.com

Keela (easier-to-use menstrual cup with pull-string): keelacup.com

Natracare (organic tampons and pads): natracare.com

Sustain Natural (organic tampons and pads, plus condoms, wipes, and lubes): sustainnatural.com

Jade and Pearl (sea sponges): jadeandpearl.com

Put a Cup in It (finding the right menstrual cup for you): putacupinit.com

BIRTH CONTROL

Bedsider: bedsider.org

Sweetening the Pill: sweeteningthepill.com

NOTES

INTRODUCTION

1. Jordan Robertson, "If Your Teen Has Menstrual Cramps, You Need to Read This," accessed May 30, 2018, drjordannd.com/if-your-teen-has-menstrual-cramps-you-need-to-read-this.
2. Anna Dahlqvist, *It's Only Blood: Shattering the Taboo of Menstruation*. London: Zed Books, 2018, 177.
3. Karen Jensen, *Women's Health Matters: The Influence of Gender on Disease*. Coquitlam: Mind Publishing, 2017.

A SHORT HISTORY OF THE CURSE

1. Abby Norman, "The Normalization of Women's Pain," interview by Amanda Laird, *The Heavy Flow Podcast*, March 26, 2018, audio, 6:02, amandalaird.ca/episode-26-the-normalization-of-women s-pain-with-abby-norman.
2. Brené Brown, "shame v. guilt," accessed June 12, 2018, brenebrown.com/blog/2013/01/14/shame-v-guilt.
3. "PandG School Programs," Procter & Gamble, accessed June 13, 2018, pgschoolprograms.com.
4. Pliny the Elder, quoted in Jennifer Weiss-Wolf, *Periods Gone Public*. New York: Arcade Publishing, 2017, 8.
5. Janice Delaney, Mary Jane Lupton, and Emily Toth, *The Curse: A Cultural History of Menstruation*. Champaign: University of Illinois Press, 1978.

6. "Menotoxin," Museum of Menstruation and Women's Health, accessed July 6, 2018, mum.org/menotox.htm.

7. Jeffrey Gettleman, "Where a Taboo Is Leading to the Deaths of Young Girls," *New York Times*, June 19, 2018, nytimes.com/2018/06/19/world/asia/nepal-women-menstruation-period.html.

8. Malaka Gharib, "Why 2015 Was the Year of the Period, and We Don't Mean Punctuation," *NPR*, December 31, 2015, npr.org/sections/health-shots/2015/12/31/460726461/why-2015-was-the-year-of-the-period-and-we-dont-mean-punctuation.

9. Anna Maltby, "The 8 Greatest Menstrual Moments of 2015," *Cosmopolitan*, October 13, 2015, cosmopolitan.com/health-fitness/news/a47609/2015-the-year-the-period-went-public.

10. Radhika Sanghani, "Instagram Deletes Woman's Period Photos — but Her Response Is Amazing," *Telegraph,* March 30, 2015, telegraph.co.uk/women/life/instagram-deletes-womans-period-photos-but-her-response-is-amazing.

11. Rupi Kaur, "period," accessed May 28, 2018, rupikaur.com/period.

12. TV By the Numbers, "Sunday Cable Ratings: 'Game of Thrones' Wins Night and 'Keeping Up With the Kardashians', 'Real Housewives of New Jersey', 'Breaking Amish', 'Mad Men' and More," accessed June 13, 2018, tvbythenumbers.zap2it.com/sdsdskdh279882992z1/sunday-cable-ratings-game-of-thrones-wins-night-keeping-up-with-the-kardashians-real-housewives-of-new-jersey-breaking-amish-mad-men-more/185649.

13. Elizabeth Yuko, "Period Pain Must Be Taken Seriously — But It Also Shouldn't Define Us," *The Establishment*, February 23, 2016, theestablishment.co/how-the-period-paradox-keeps-women-down-6b956d7fcb10.

14. Emma Sagner, "More States Move to End 'Tampon Tax' That's Seen as Discriminating Against Women,' *NPR*, March 25, 2018, npr.org/2018/03/25/564580736/more-states-move-to-end-tampon-tax-that-s-seen-as-discriminating-against-women.

15. Bobel, interview, May 24, 2018.

16. S.L. Vostral, "Rely and Toxic Shock Syndrome: A Technological Health Crisis," *The Yale Journal of Biology and Medicine* 84, no. 4. (2011): 447–59, ncbi.nlm.nih.gov/pmc/articles/PMC3238331.

17. "Welcome to #periodpositive," #periodpositive, accessed July 16, 2018, periodpositive.com.

18. Irene Whittaker-Cumming, email to author, July 18, 2018.

19. "Treatments for Menstrual Cramps Throughout History," Museum of Health Care, accessed June 23 2018, museumofhealthcare. wordpress.com/2015/09/17/treatments-for-menstrual-cramps-throughout-history/#_ftn4.

20. Elizabeth Yuko, "Period Pain Must Be Taken Seriously — But It Also Shouldn't Define Us," *The Establishment*, February 23, 2016, theestablishment.co/how-the-period-paradox-keeps-women-down-6b956d7fcb10.

21. L. Culley, C. Law, N. Hudson, H. Mitchell, E. Denny, N. Raine-Fenning, "A Qualitative Study of the Impact of Endometriosis on Male Partners," *Human Reproduction* 32, no. 8 (August 1, 2017): 1667–73, doi.org/10.1093/humrep/dex221.

22. S. Iacovides, I. Avidon, and FC Baker, "What We Know About Primary Dysmenorrhea Today: A Critical Review," *Human Reproduction Update* 21, no. 6 (2015): 762–78, doi:10.1093/humupd/dmv039, ncbi.nlm.nih.gov/pubmed/26346058.

23. Abby Norman, "The Normalization of Women's Pain," interview by Amanda Laird, *The Heavy Flow Podcast*, March 26, 2018, audio, 14:38, amandalaird.ca/episode-26-the-normalization-of-womens-pain-with-abby-norman.

24. "Pain Is Real and Shouldn't Be Dismissed," Endometriosis UK, accessed July 9, 2018, endometriosis-uk.org/awareness-week-2014.

25. Kenneth Miller, "How Health Care Fails Women," *Prevention*, July 2, 2018, prevention.com/health/a22022580/how-health-care-fails-women.

26. The poll was ongoing.

27. Kenneth Miller, "How Health Care Fails Women," *Prevention*, July 2, 2018, prevention.com/health/a22022580/how-health-care-fails-women.

28. Joe Fassler, "How Doctors Take Women's Pain Less Seriously," *The Atlantic*, October 15, 2015, theatlantic.com/health/archive/2015/10/emergency-room-wait-times-sexism/410515.

29. Diane E. Hoffman and Anita J. Tarzian, "The Girl Who Cried Pain: A Bias Against Women in the Treatment of Pain," *Journal of Law, Medicine and Ethics* 29 (2001):13–27, ssrn.com/abstract=383803.

30. M.E. McPherson and L. Korfine, "Menstruation Across Time: Menarche, Menstrual Attitudes, Experiences, and Behaviors," *Women's Health Issues* 14, no. 6 (2004): 193–200, ncbi.nlm.nih.gov/pubmed/15589769.

31. J. Brooks-Gunn and D.N. Ruble, "The Development of Menstrual-Related Beliefs and Behaviors During Early Adolescence," *Child Development* 53, no. 6 (1982): 1567–77, ncbi.nlm.nih.gov/pubmed/7172782.

32. R.K. Jones, "Beyond Birth Control: The Overlooked Benefits of Oral Contraceptive Pills," New York: Guttmacher Institute, 2011. guttmacher.org/sites/default/files/report_pdf/beyond-birth-control.pdf.

33. Jonathan Eig, "The Team That Invented the Birth Control Pill," *The Atlantic*, accessed October 2, 108, theatlantic.com/health/archive/2014/10/the-team-that-invented-the-birth-control-pill/380684/.

34. Susan Rako, M.D., *The Blessings of the Curse: No More Periods?* Place: iUniverse, Inc., 2006.

35. Rachel Morris, "What It Really Takes to Get Pregnant After Birth Control," *Parents*, accessed June 24, 2018, parents.com/getting-pregnant/fertility/boostwhat-it-really-takes-to-get-pregnant-after-birth-control.

36. Lisa Hendrickson-Jack, "Using Fertility Awareness to Claim the Power of the Menstrual Cycle," interview by Amanda Laird, *The Heavy Flow Podcast*, March 1, 2018, audio, 27:47, amandalaird.ca/episode-22-using-fertility-awareness-to-claim-the-power-of-the-menstrual-cycle-with-lisa-hendrickson-jack/.

37. Rae Ellen Bichell, "Average Age of First-Time Moms Keeps Climbing in the U.S.," *NPR*, January 14, 2016, npr.org/sections/health-shots/2016/01/14/462816458/average-age-of-first-time-moms-keeps-climbing-in-the-u-s.

38. Amy Sutherland, email to author, July 6, 2018.

CHAPTER 1: GETTING TO KNOW YOUR BODY

1. "Global Health Observatory (GHO) Data," World Health Organization, accessed June 18, 2018, who.int/gho/mortality_burden_disease/life_tables/situation_trends/en.

2. Laura Wershler, "Increasing Body Literacy with Fertility Awareness | Health Benefits of Regular Ovulation | Feminism and the Pill," interview by Lisa Hendrickson-Jack, *The Fertility Friday Podcast*, July 31, 2015, audio, 19:56, fertilityfriday.com/laurawershler.

3. "Menstrual Cycle Health," Justisse Healthworks for Women, accessed June 24, 2018, justisse.ca/index.php/pages/page/menstrual-cycle-health.

4. Jerilynn C. Prior, "Preventive Powers of Ovulation and Progesterone," Centre for Menstrual Cycle and Ovulation Research, accessed May 28, 2018, cemcor.ca/files/uploads/6_Ovulation_and_Breast_Health.pdf.

5. Danni Li, Christine L. Hitchcock, Susan I. Barr, Tricia Yu, and Jerilynn C. Prior, "Negative Spinal Bone Mineral Density Changes and Subclinical Ovulatory Disturbances — Prospective Data in Healthy Premenopausal Women with Regular Menstrual Cycles," *Epidemiologic Reviews* 36, no. 1 (2014): 137–47, doi: 10.1093/epirev/mxt012, cemcor.ca/sites/default/files/uploads/Li%202013%20Negative%20BMD...ovulatory%20disturbances%20Epidemiol%20Rev.pdf.

6. Jerilynn C. Prior, "Progesterone Within Ovulatory Menstrual Cycles Needed for Cardiovascular Protection: An Evidence-Based Hypothesis," *Journal of Restorative Medicine* 3, no. 1 (2014): 85–103, cemcor.ca/sites/default/files/uploads/Prior%202014%20Progesterone...%20needed...%20CV%20protection...%20J%20Restor%20Med.pdf.

CHAPTER 2: UNDERSTANDING THE MENSTRUAL CYCLE

1. "Menstruation in Girls and Adolescents: Using the Menstrual Cycle as a Vital Sign," American College of Obstetricians and Gynecologists, December 2015, acog.org/Clinical-Guidance-and-Publications/Committee-Opinions/Committee-on-Adolescent-Health-Care/Menstruation-in-Girls-and-Adolescents-Using-the-Menstrual-Cycle-as-a-Vital-Sign.

2. "Menstrual Cycle Health," Justisse Healthworks for Women, accessed June 24, 2018, justisse.ca/index.php/pages/page/menstrual-cycle-health.

3. "Vital Signs," *Dictionary.com*, accessed August 26, 2018, dictionary. com/browse/vital-signs?s=t.

4. "What Is Osteoporosis?" Osteoporosis, accessed June 24, 2018, osteoporosis.ca/about-the-disease/what-is-osteoporosis.

5. G.I. Smith, et al., "Testosterone and Progesterone, But Not Estradiol, Stimulate Muscle Protein Synthesis in Postmenopausal Women," *Journal of Clinical Endocrinology and Metabolism* 99, no. 1 (2014): 256–65, doi:10.1210/jc.2013-2835, ncbi.nlm.nih.gov/pmc/articles/ PMC3879672.

6. "New Study Highlights Progesterone Benefit for Breast Cancer," *Health Canal*, June 24, 2016, healthcanal.com/cancers/breast-cancer/ 73605-new-study-highlights-progesterone-benefit-for-breast-cancer. html.

7. Jerilynn C. Prior, "Preventive Powers of Ovulation and Progesterone," Centre for Menstrual Cycle and Ovulation Research, accessed May 28, 2018, cemcor.ca/files/uploads/6_Ovulation_and_Breast_Health.pdf.

8. "Progesterone and the Nervous System/Brain," Women in Balance Institute, National University of Natural Medicine, accessed July 15, 2018, womeninbalance.org/resources-research/ progesterone-and-the-nervous-systembrain.

9. Claudia Valeggia, "Until the Baby Can Walk," interview by Kate Clancy, *Period.*, December 15, 2017, 26:26, audio, kateclancy.com/ period18.

10. "Menopause," The Centre for Menstrual Cycle and Ovulation Research, accessed May 29, 2018, cemcor.ubc.ca/resources/life-phases/ menopause.

CHAPTER 3: FINDING YOUR NORMAL

1. Laura Wershler, "#bodyliteracy: A Hashtag, a Title, a Meme?" *Menstruation Matters*, June 28, 2012, menstruationresearch. org/2012/06/28/bodyliteracy-a-hashtag-a-title-a-meme.

2. "Scientific Basis," Justisse Healthworks for Women, accessed July 8, 2018, 13:14, justisse.ca/index.php/pages/page/justisse-scientific-basis.

3. "Menstrual Cycle Health," Justisse Healthworks for Women, accessed June 24, 2018, justisse.ca/index.php/pages/page/menstrual-cycle-health.

4.   "Scientific Basis," Justisse Healthworks for Women, accessed July 8, 2018, justisse.ca/index.php/pages/page/justisse-scientific-basis.

CHAPTER 4: WHEN GOOD PERIODS GO BAD

1.   Elizabeth Yuko, "Period Pain Must Be Taken Seriously — But It Also Shouldn't Define Us," *The Establishment*, February 23, 2016, theestablishment.co/how-the-period-paradox-keeps-women-down-6b956d7fcb10.

2.   Jordan Robertson, "PMS: Why You Shouldn't Be Tested," *Integrative Medicine Podcast*, May 13, 2018, audio, 8:40, drjordannd.com/podcast/podcast-2-pms-why-you-shouldnt-be-tested.

3.   Phyllis A. Balch, CNC, *Prescription for Nutritional Healing*, Fifth Edition. New York: Avery, 2010.

4.   P.M.S. O'Brien, et al., "Towards a Consensus on Diagnostic Criteria, Measurement and Trial Design of the Premenstrual Disorders: The ISPMD Montreal Consensus," *Archives of Women's Mental Health* 14, no. 1 (2011): 13–21. doi:10.1007/s00737-010-0201-3, ncbi.nlm.nih.gov/pmc/articles/PMC4134928.

5.   Jordan Robertson, "PMS: Why You Shouldn't Be Tested," *Integrative Medicine Podcast*, May 13, 2018, audio, 8:40, drjordannd.com/podcast/podcast-2-pms-why-you-shouldnt-be-tested.

6.   Phyllis A. Balch, CNC, *Prescription for Nutritional Healing*, Fifth Edition. New York: Avery, 2010.

7.   "Heavy Menstrual Bleeding," Alignment Monkey, November 17, 2014, alignmentmonkey.nurturance.net/2014/heavy-menstrual-bleeding.

8.   H. Ju, M. Jones, and G. Mishra, "The Prevalence and Risk Factors of Dysmenorrhea," *Epidemiol Review* 36 (2014): 104–13. doi: 10.1093/epirev/mxt009, ncbi.nlm.nih.gov/pubmed/24284871.

9.   "Cramps and Painful Periods," Centre for Menstrual Cycle and Ovulation Research, accessed May 31, 2018, cemcor.ubc.ca/resources/topics/cramps-and-painful-periods.

10. E.A. MacGregor, J. Brandes, A. Eikermann, R. Giammarco, "Impact of Migraine on Patients and Their Families: The Migraine and Zolmitriptan Evaluation (MAZE) Survey — Phase III," *Current Medical Research and Opinion* 20, no. 7 (2004): 1143–50, ncbi.nlm.nih.gov/pubmed/15265259.

11. Christiane Northrup, M.D., *Women's Bodies, Women's Wisdom: Creating Physical and Emotional Health and Healing*, Revised and Updated. New York: Bantam Books, 2010.

12. Francis Hutchins, quoted in C. Northrup, M.D., *Women's Bodies, Women's Wisdom*.

13. Lara N.D. Briden, *Period Repair Manual: Natural Treatment for Better Hormones and Better Periods*, Second Edition. New Zealand: Author, 2017.

CHAPTER 5: YOUR PERIOD QUESTIONS ANSWERED

1. Breanne Fahs, Jax Gonzalez, Rose Coursey, and Stephanie Robinson-Cestaro, "Cycling Together: Menstrual Synchrony as a Projection of Gendered Solidarity," *Women's Reproductive Health* 1 (2014): 90–105. doi:10.1080/23293691.2014.966029, academia.edu/21697594/Cycling_Together_Menstrual_Synchrony_as_a_Projection_of_Gendered_Solidarity.

2. F. Hollwich and B. Dieckhues, "The Effect of Natural and Artificial Light via the Eye on the Hormonal and Metabolic Balance of Animal and Man," *Ophthalmologica* 180, no. 4 (1980): 188–97, ncbi.nlm.nih.gov/pubmed/6255392.

3. Beverly I. Strassmann, "The Biology of Menstruation in Homo Sapiens: Total Lifetime Menses, Fecundity, and Nonsynchrony in Natural-Fertility Population," *Current Anthropology* 38, no. 1 (1997): 123–29, journals.uchicago.edu/doi/10.1086/204592.

CHAPTER 7: THE NUTRITION APPROACH TO PERIOD CARE

1. J. K. Kiecolt-Glaster, et al., "Depression, Daily Stressors and Inflammatory Responses to High-Fat Meals: When Stress Overrides Healthier Food Choices," *Molecular Psychiatry* 22 (2017): 476–82, nature.com/articles/mp2016149.

CHAPTER 8: FOODS FOR SUPPORTING HORMONAL HEALTH

1. S.L. Gorbach and B.R. Goldin, "Diet and the Excretion and Enterohepatic Cycling of Estrogens," *Preventative Medicine* 16, no. 4 (1987): 525–31, ncbi.nlm.nih.gov/pubmed/3628202.

2. H.B. Patisaul and W. Jefferson, "The Pros and Cons of Phytoestrogens," *Frontiers in Neuroendocrinology* 31, no. 4 (2010): 400–19. doi:10.1016/j.yfrne.2010.03.003, ncbi.nlm.nih.gov/pmc/articles/PMC3074428.

3. J.M. Choi, et al., "Increased Prevalence of Celiac Disease in Patients with Unexplained Infertility in the United States," *Journal of Reproductive Medicine* 56, no. 5–6 (2011): 199–203, ncbi.nlm.nih.gov/pubmed/21682114.

4. M. Marziali, M. Venza, S. Lazzaro, A. Lazzaro, C. Micossi, and V.M. Stolfi, "Gluten-free Diet: A New Strategy for Management of Painful Endometriosis Related Symptoms?" *Minerva Chichurgia* 67, no. 6 (2012): 499–504, ncbi.nlm.nih.gov/pubmed/23334113.

5. "How the Products in Your Home Affect Your Fertility," *Green at Home*, accessed June 26, 2018, greenathome.ca/wp-content/uploads/2017/09/Your-Home-and-Your-Health-Fertility-Factsheet.pdf.

6. "Shopper's Guide to Pesticides in Produce™," EWG Home, accessed May 17, 2018, ewg.org/foodnews.

7. Jessica Murnane, "Endometriosis and Eating Plants for Self Care," interview by Amanda Laird, *The Heavy Flow Podcast*, audio, October 12, 2017, 9:11, amandalaird.ca/episode-06-endometriosis-eating-plants-for-self-care-with-jessica-murnane.

CHAPTER 9: STRESS AND YOUR MENSTRUAL CYCLE

1. Lara N.D. Briden, *Period Repair Manual: Natural Treatment for Better Hormones and Better Periods*, Second Edition. New Zealand: Author, 2017.

CHAPTER 10: OTHER LIFESTYLE FACTORS FOR BETTER PERIODS

1. Z. Mohebbi Dehnavi, F. Jafarnejad, and S. Sadeghi Goghary, "The Effect of 8 Weeks Aerobic Exercise on Severity of Physical Symptoms of Premenstrual Syndrome: A Clinical Trial Study," *BMC Womens Health* 19, no. 1 (2018): 80, doi:10.1186/s12905-018-0565-5, ncbi. nlm.nih.gov/pubmed/29855308.

2. "Exposures Add Up — Survey Results," EWG's Skin Deep® Cosmetics Database, accessed July 11, 2018, ewg.org/skindeep/2004/06/15/ exposures-add-up-survey-results/#.W0YVCNhKiCQ.

3. K. Sieja and J. von Mach-Szczypiński, "Health Effect of Chronic Exposure to Carbon Disulfide (C2) on Women Employed in Viscose Industry," *Medycyna Pracy* 69, no. 3 (2018): 329–35. doi:10.13075/ mp.5893.00600, ncbi.nlm.nih.gov/pubmed/29171550.

4. Louis Nonfoux, et al., "Impact of Currently Marketed Tampons and Menstrual Cups on Staphylococcus Aureus Growth and TSST-1 Production in Vitro," *Applied and Environmental Microbiology* April 20, 2018, doi:10.1128/AEM.00351-18, aem.asm.org/content/ early/2018/04/02/AEM.00351-18.abstract.

5. M.A. Mitchell, S. Bisch, S. Arntfield, and S.M. Hosseini-Moghaddam, "A Confirmed Case of Toxic Shock Syndrome Associated with the Use of a Menstrual Cup," *The Canadian Journal of Infectious Diseases and Medical Microbiology* 26, no. 4 (2015): 218–20, ncbi.nlm.nih. gov/pmc/articles/PMC4556184.

CHAPTER 11: MANAGING YOUR PERIOD PAIN

1. Alice Park, "The Ibuprofen Risks You Need to Know," *Time*, April 20, 2017, ime.com/4746319/ibuprofen-painkillers-risks.

2. K.P. Hill, M.D. Palastro, B. Johnson, and J.W. Ditre, "Cannabis and Pain: A Clinical Review," *Cannabis and Cannabinoid Research* 2, no. 1 (2017): 96–104, doi:10.1089/can.2017.0017, ncbi.nlm.nih.gov/ pmc/articles/PMC5549367.

3. Maya Elisabeth, "Medical Marijuana (CBD, Edibles, and Topicals) Explained," interview with Jessica Murnane, *One Part Podcast*, audio, October 4, 2017, 49:07, jessicamurnane.com/ medical-marijuana-cbd-edibles-and-topicals-explained.

4. M.Y. Dawood and J. Ramos, "Transcutaneous Electrical Nerve Stimulation (TENS) for the Treatment of Primary Dysmenorrhea: A Randomized Crossover Comparison with Placebo TENS and Ibuprofen," *Obstetrics & Gynecology* 75, no. 4 (1990): 656–60, ncbi. nlm.nih.gov/pubmed/2179780.

CHAPTER 12: HORMONAL HEALTH AFTER BIRTH CONTROL

1. Ross Pelton, *The Pill Problem: How to Protect Your Health from the Side Effects of Oral Contraceptives.* BookBaby, 2013.

2. Jolene Brighten, "Post-Birth Control Syndrome and How to Heal Now," accessed June 19, 2018, drbrighten.com/post-birth-control-syndrome.

CHAPTER 13: TUNING IN TO YOUR CYCLE

1. J. Brooks-Gunn and D.N. Ruble, "The Development of Menstrual-Related Beliefs and Behaviors during Early Adolescence," *Child Development* 53, no. 6 (1982): 1567–77, ncbi.nlm.nih.gov/ pubmed/7172782.

CHAPTER 14: WORKING WITH, NOT AGAINST, YOUR HORMONES

1. Alisa Vitti, *WomanCode: Perfect Your Cycle, Amplify Your Fertility, Supercharge Your Sex Drive, and Become a Power Source.* New York: HarperCollins, 2013.

CHAPTER 15: TALKING TO THE NEXT GENERATION

1. Amy Sutherland, email to author, July 6, 2018.

INDEX

Book Credits

Acquiring Editor: Margaret Bryant
Developmental Editor: Allison Hirst
Project Editor: Elena Radic
Copy Editor: Heather Bean
Proofreader: Emma Warnken Johnson

Cover Designer: Laura Boyle
Interior Designer: Sophie Paas-Lang

Publicist: Tabassum Siddiqui

Dundurn

Publisher: J. Kirk Howard
Vice-President: Carl A. Brand
Editorial Director: Kathryn Lane
Artistic Director: Laura Boyle
Production Manager: Rudi Garcia
Publicity Manager: Michelle Melski
Manager, Accounting and Technical Services: Livio Copetti

Editorial: Allison Hirst, Dominic Farrell, Jenny McWha,
Rachel Spence, Elena Radic, Melissa Kawaguchi

Marketing and Publicity: Kendra Martin, Elham Ali,
Tabassum Siddiqui, Heather McLeod

Design and Production: Sophie Paas-Lang

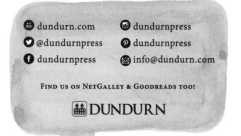

dundurn.com   dundurnpress
@dundurnpress   dundurnpress
dundurnpress   info@dundurn.com

FIND US ON NETGALLEY & GOODREADS TOO!

DUNDURN